How to Manage Your GP Practice

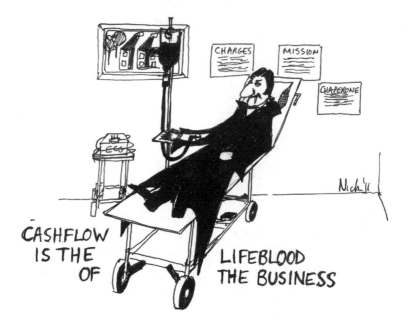

How to Manage Your GP Practice

Farine Clarke and Laurence Slavin

Illustrated by Nick Clarke

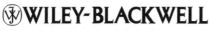

WILEY-BLACKWELL

A John Wiley & Sons, Ltd., Publication

BMJ|Books

This edition first published 2012 © 2012 by John Wiley & Sons, Ltd.

BMJ Books is an imprint of BMJ Publishing Group Limited, used under licence by Blackwell Publishing which was acquired by John Wiley & Sons in February 2007. Blackwell's publishing programme has been merged with Wiley's global Scientific, Technical and Medical business to form Wiley-Blackwell.

Registered office: John Wiley & Sons, Ltd, The Atrium, Southern Gate, Chichester, West Sussex, PO19 8SQ, UK

Editorial offices: 9600 Garsington Road, Oxford, OX4 2DQ, UK
The Atrium, Southern Gate, Chichester, West Sussex, PO19 8SQ, UK
111 River Street, Hoboken, NJ 07030-5774, USA

For details of our global editorial offices, for customer services and for information about how to apply for permission to reuse the copyright material in this book please see our website at www.wiley.com/wiley-blackwell

The right of the author to be identified as the author of this work has been asserted in accordance with the UK Copyright, Designs and Patents Act 1988.

Library of Congress Cataloging-in-Publication Data

Clarke, Farine.
How to manage your GP practice / by Farine Clarke and Laurence Slavin.
p. ; cm.
Includes index.
ISBN 978-0-470-65784-3 (pbk.)
1. Family medicine–Practice. I. Slavin, Laurence. II. Title.
[DNLM: 1. Practice Management, Medical–organization & administration–Great Britain. 2. General Practice–organization & administration–Great Britain. 3. State Medicine–Great Britain. W 80]
R729.5.G4C63 2011
610.68–dc23

2011020602

A catalogue record for this book is available from the British Library.

This book is published in the following electronic formats: ePDF 9781119959533; Wiley Online Library 9781119959564; ePub 9781119959540

Set in 9.5/12pt Minion by Thomson Digital, Noida, India
Printed and bound in Malaysia by Vivar Printing Sdn Bhd

1   2012

Contents

Preface, vii

Chapter 1: The business as an organism, 1

Chapter 2: The challenge that is staff, 17

Chapter 3: Basic practice accounting, 37

Chapter 4: Budgeting, 73

Chapter 5: Choosing the right operational model for the practice, 81

Chapter 6: Business growth, 87

Chapter 7: Planning for the exit, 99

Chapter 8: Ten questions answered, 113

Chapter 9: Thou shalt . . . thou shalt not!, 125

Appendix 1: Useful contacts, 127

Appendix 2: Full set of practice accounts, 129

Index, 143

Preface

Doctors practice medicine to treat patients. If they had wanted to be business people or managers, they would have done MBAs and entered commerce; all of this is true. But GPs in partnerships today have to be all things to all people: they have to make sure their patients receive rapid and appropriate treatment, and they also have to ensure their practices remain healthy. To achieve this, partners need to have as advanced an understanding of what it takes to run a small business as they do to manage complex patients. Just as the pressure on patient care has increased beyond recognition in recent decades, so has the pressure on small business to demonstrate 'best practice'. Doctors need to be prepared for a host of new threats to their practice, from staff litigation which is increasing at a rate reminiscent to that of medico-legal cases in recent years, to the rules and regulations accompanying European legislation, and their impact on practice management. All of this comes on top of the basic need for partners to make sufficient profit to pay themselves and their staff appropriately, and to grow and develop their practices as they wish.

This book sprang from a conversation between the authors about the lack of credible practical information for doctors and the need to arm GPs or private practitioners with the right information to achieve success. It was written in response to a request from doctors for a clear, accessible book detailing the most useful financial and business information for them. They did not want a lecture or to be blinded by management jargon, but wanted straightforward practical information, presented using real-life examples to illustrate the salient points. In short, a book which they could draw on for advice, but with which they could easily relate. The authors believe and hope that this is such a book.

Farine Clarke qualified from St George's Hospital Medical School, London in 1986 and completed the St Helier hospital GP vocational Training Scheme. She decided to pursue a career in publishing where she worked first on *Pulse* and then on *GP* as editor and editorial director. She was promoted through the ranks to managing director firstly at Haymarket Medical Ltd, where she was responsible for *GP*, *Medeconomics* and *MIMS*, and then at Archant Specialist Ltd, where she ran 15 consumer magazines, ranging from *Photography Monthly* to *The English Garden*. In her roles as managing director and main board director, Farine was responsible for the profit and loss, staff management, product development and expansion of the companies she ran, both in the United Kingdom and overseas. Farine feels strongly that doctors have the skills to manage complex businesses, but have not always received the most appropriate training and do not always have access to the type of information which would help them the most. Farine is married to Nick Clarke, a consultant old age psychiatrist. They have one son and live in East Sussex.

Laurence Slavin is a chartered accountant and has been a partner with the London based firm Ramsay Brown and Partners for more than 20 years. His practice specialises in advising and working with GPs and GP practices. Currently Laurence's practice has more than 500 GP practices on their books and advises more than 2,500 GPs. Laurence was a specialist advisor to the former NHS Management Executive for ten years, and served as an advisor to the Department of Health sitting on the Pensions Sub-committee during the negotiations over the 2004 New Contract. Since 1989 he has been writing a regular column in *GP* magazine and *Medeconomics*, advising GPs on financial and practice management. Laurence lectures regularly to GPs, practice managers and GP registrars on matters of personal and practice finance in both the United Kingdom and overseas. He has appeared as an expert witness in a number of legal civil actions involving GPs. Laurence is married to a GP and has four children and a giant schnauzer named Hector.

Chapter 1 **The business as an organism**

The Green practice used to be a successful five-partner practice led for many years by the two senior partners, whose main aim was to provide excellent clinical service. As a result the practice expanded rapidly, although the partners showed little interest in the accounts, referring to them as 'Monopoly money'. At their annual meeting the accountant expressed concern that profits were falling faster than expected. Instead of trying to get to the root of this downward pressure on profits, the partners remained disinterested and continued with their usual drawings. At the following annual meeting, one of the senior partners revealed that the practice funds were exhausted and the bank had recalled the existing overdraft, with no prospect of extending a new one, due to the current economic climate. As a result the partners had to repay six months' drawings and accept reduced continuing drawings. Two partners subsequently resigned. Not surprisingly, the Green practice is now a shadow of its former self.

Dr Stevens was one of a four-partner GP practice in Northampton. Instead of saving money each month to pay his tax, he borrowed the funds whenever this payment was due. In January 2009 he requested the usual finance from his bank manager, but this year, as a result of the economic downturn, the bank refused. Dr Stevens ignored the demands and letters from HMRC and was ultimately bankrupted by them. As a result, he was expelled from his partnership because, by law, he could not be a principal and a bankrupt. Dr Stevens was employed as a salaried GP before finally being made redundant.

The two examples above may seem extreme, but they are both real-life cases, and demonstrate issues which can, to a greater or lesser degree, affect many GPs. In this book the authors will use a range of anecdotes like these to illustrate what it takes to run a successful practice as well as highlighting the pitfalls along the way. The examples given may push the boundaries of

How to Manage Your GP Practice, First Edition. Farine Clarke and Laurence Slavin.
© 2012 John Wiley & Sons, Ltd. Published 2012 by John Wiley & Sons, Ltd.

credibility, but they are all genuine cases. The names and locations have been changed to preserve anonymity. By drawing on examples in other business disciplines, we aim to arm GPs with additional tools to make the most of their practices. This book explains best practice with regard to accounts, partnerships, staff and competition, whichever government is in power and whatever changes are taking place in the NHS, from the dissolution of primary care trusts (PCTs) to the creation of consortia. The business skills detailed here are eminently transferable across disciplines and economic conditions. GPs can operate as sole traders, partners in a partnership or directors of a limited company, and although the text refers to partners the issues will apply to all roles. Most importantly this book is definitely not a 'GPs *should* do this' or 'GPs *must* do that' title: we feel there is quite enough lecturing in other publications. Instead we hope that, as a specialist GP accountant who has advised thousands of GP practices for many years, and a former GP with decades of experience running commercial businesses at main board level, we have valuable expertise to share with colleagues. Most of all, we hope GPs will enjoy reading this book, benefit from those chapters which are most relevant to them and feel far better informed and equipped at the end of it than they did at the beginning.

Dirty money or life blood?

To many GPs, 'money' is a dirty word in the context of professional practice. This is perfectly understandable: after all, the vast majority have grown up in the NHS where best clinical practice, not revenue and profit, governs their professionalism. Even those who eventually work in private practice always put their patients before the profit, and the authors would not have it any other way. However, a healthy practice is not simply one which treats its patients successfully. Indeed a healthy practice, like any commercial business, will be more successful if it manages all aspects of its being, including its staff, buildings, contracts, relationships and, yes, finances at optimum levels. Only by doing this effectively can a practice truly develop, grow and serve its patients to its full potential.

Your practice is a living, breathing organism: it has objectives and purpose, but it also needs a life force to support it. Money represents the blood circulating through the practice: cut off the supply and the practice will die. Ensure nothing is blocking or reducing the circulation and the practice will thrive.

What do we mean by money? When someone says they are making lots of money we assume they are making profits. Conversely, when they say they are not making money we assume they are unable to pay their debts, which means, they are insolvent. In this context, money has two meanings, profitability and solvency, and it is vital to understand the difference to maintain a healthy practice. A healthy practice will be profitable and solvent.

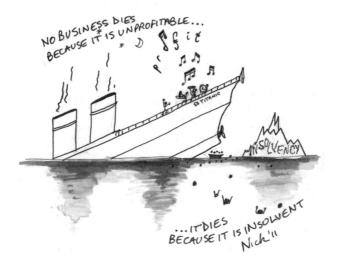

An unhealthy practice will be profitable and insolvent, or unprofitable and solvent, or, worst of all, unprofitable and insolvent.

No business dies because it is unprofitable; it dies because it is insolvent. If, for example, it is unprofitable but is still solvent, that is, it can still raise funds,

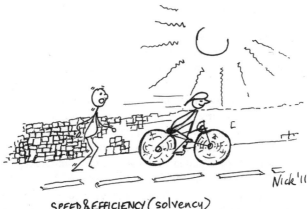

it is sick, but it is not dead. However, if that business has a number of creditors and the bank calls in its overdraft facility, then it will switch from being unprofitable and solvent to unprofitable and insolvent, at which point it *will* die. This is what happened to the Green practice. If a company cannot pay its bills, a creditor can petition for it to be put into liquidation. For professional partnerships, unless they operate as a limited company, the equivalent of liquidation is the bankruptcy of a partner. Both liquidation and bankruptcy have catastrophic results. In the case of the Green practice, the problem only became critical when the bank withdrew the overdraft, effectively cutting off the practice's blood supply and rendering it insolvent. In Dr Stevens' case, it ended a successful medical career and added considerable tensions to his private life.

The keys to success

In a successful practice, the following key components work together in harmony:
- Vision
- Direction
- Decision making
- Partnership
- Staff
- Premises
- Service
- Patients

Your vision or mine?

Every component of a successful practice stems from its vision. By vision we mean the aims and targets for that practice and its partners. These may be long term, for example doubling the practice size over the next five years through a combination of acquisition and organic growth. Or they may be short term, for example introducing a specialist facility or extending an existing building within six months. Of course many practices will have a combination of long and short term visions, and, as with any business, these will require review and revision from time to time, depending on progress and changing circumstances. There are no hard and fast rules governing visions, except perhaps that they should be shared and documented. The worst thing would be for three partners in a practice to be dreaming of three quite different aims in isolation in their individual consulting rooms. This makes the likelihood of success rather slim.

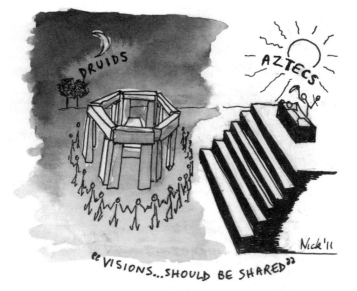

"VISIONS...SHOULD BE SHARED"

The practice vision may come from all the partners or just one person. But, if there is nobody with vision, the business will be devoid of direction, and without a direction the partners and staff will work in a vacuum, unable to prioritise and coordinate with each other to achieve the same goals. Therefore every practice will benefit from identifying those individuals who are visionary, without automatically assuming that this person is the senior partner:

Dr Collins, aged 43, and Dr Graham, aged 29, were part of a well respected, successful surgery that was run by Dr Smythe, an autocratic but extremely talented senior partner. When Dr Smythe died suddenly aged 55, Dr Collins automatically took over the 'senior' role including the financial and directional responsibilities. He was preoccupied with detail, spending extraordinary amounts of time preparing schedules of the practice expenses, and analysing invoices from each and every supplier. He was troubled by making claims to the PCT unless he was satisfied the content was complete and correct, and referenced back to the original work done in the practice. But Dr Collins never stepped back to take a strategic, long term view of his practice. At the same time Dr Graham generated 80% of the practice work. Within a year of Dr Smythe's death, the practice was in debt and unable to service its bank overdraft. Dr Graham, who was unaware of the severity of the situation, was horrified when the bank asked both partners to take out second mortgages on their homes. He held an emergency meeting with the bank manager in which he explained how the practice had been working. As a result, he dissolved the partnership and set up on his own without a second mortgage. Dr Graham now runs a successful practice with two new partners, while Dr Collins barely manages to stay afloat.

Vision alone is not enough for success. Indeed, those without vision will still have very important qualities which are vital for a practice. Success requires a balance of partners, each playing to their individual strengths. A business full of visionaries will fail if it is unable to manage those visions when they become reality:

The Black practice had four visionary partners and an equally visionary manager. As a team, they had no difficulty agreeing and executing their aims, meaning the practice expanded rapidly by taking over a number of local surgeries. Their size doubled, but their profits fell. When this was investigated, it turned out that none of the partners, or the practice manager, took an active interest in running the new surgeries post acquisition. They had not even visited any of the new sites, which were left to manage themselves. No effort was made to boost morale or control costs. In the end, the acquired practices were disbanded and the patients dispersed to neighbouring surgeries.

When commercial companies make acquisitions, they go through a vigorous process involving business plans, due diligence and, as importantly, a post-acquisition consolidation plan. In these plans the methods by which the new business will be incorporated into the existing one are set out in detail. Cost savings are identified together with the timescale for executing them, as well as opportunities for further growth. Above all, the individuals who will carry out the consolidation process are clearly identified and charged with this responsibility. This is because what can be achieved on paper is often different when it comes to the reality of encouraging new and old staff with differing working practices to work together to deliver the plans. GPs may be a unique group, but the principles governing the consolidation of two companies are the same for any business.

You go in that direction and I'll go . . . !

All practices both have and need a direction. A practice may go round in circles, but it still has a direction, albeit one which drains its energy without taking it forward.

Everyone involved in the practice needs to know where it is going and why it is going there, together with some idea of the method and timescale.

Mission statements are somewhat clichéd, but nevertheless without direction a practice will never achieve its goals:

Partners at the Blue practice had two issues: they owed their ex-partner Dr Hill £100,000 to buy her out of the premises, and they also wanted to expand their activities. As a result they swung from negotiating with Dr Hill to searching for new premises, but never in a co-ordinated fashion. The partners remained stuck in this hopeless position for more than five years without resolution: Dr Hill continued to demand her money, while the premises were increasingly unsuitable and limiting. If the partners had written a plan, together with a realistic timetable to achieve both aims, they would have avoided this impasse.

Can we decide who's making the decisions?

Even when it appears to be going nowhere, a business does not stand still. Therefore effective decision making and subsequent active management are key to ensuring a practice runs smoothly. All partners in a partnership will benefit from an agreed decision making process with a corresponding written protocol which has been incorporated into the partnership agreement. For limited companies, the directors' powers are set out in the Articles of Association while the shareholders work within the protocols set out in the Shareholders Agreement. At first sight this might appear to be overkill, but doing this in advance, when there is not a pressing issue to deal with, really can help the partners and directors when difficult decisions do need to be made. The protocol can cover a range of situations from decisions which can readily be delegated to one individual to those requiring consideration by all the individuals involved with the business. Similarly non-contentious issues like setting staff pay rises may be decided by a majority vote, while more significant ones such as taking on a new partner, appointing a new practice manager or dismissing a member of staff may require unanimous agreement.

It is important to get the right balance into the agreement so that the protocol is neither too loose nor too restrictive, and works for the practice overall. If all decisions require unanimous consensus by all partners, an unnecessary amount of energy will be spent discussing each one and simple problems will become complicated. Far better for critical decisions to be made by all partners and operational ones reached by a simple majority. Partnership dynamics, like boardroom dynamics, are complicated and at times uncomfortable. Furthermore GPs do not like to be seen to disagree with colleagues, but if the protocols are clear and every partner has signed up to them in advance, it is far easier for an individual who finds themselves outvoted on a particular issue to not take it personally.

Box 1.1 Partnership decision grid

	Unanimous	Majority	Delegated
Appointing a new partner	x		
Appointing or dismissing staff	x		
Engaging in another business activity	x		
Forgiving a debt >£1,000	x	x	
Deciding to charge, sublet, assign, sell, transfer, lease or mortgage any practice asset	x		
Approving an expenditure <£500			x
expenditure >£5,000		x	
Approving an expenditure >£50,000	x		

Senior staff as well as partners make decisions in the practice. This means the parameters within which they are expected to function must be made clear at the outset as failing to do so can have disastrous results:

The six-partner Lavender practice in East London asked their accountant to investigate why the partnership was increasingly overdrawn. He duly prepared and analysed the year to date accounts and was surprised to find the staff costs were more than 90% of the total practice income. This was before the partners' drawings and contrasted sharply with most GP partnerships, where staff costs account for around 30% of the total practice income.

Further investigation revealed that the practice manager had been paying herself overtime as well as employing her husband and sister at generous hourly rates. On discovering this, the partners dismissed her immediately. Her response was to sue them for unfair dismissal, claiming that her instructions on employment were to deal with problems and ensure the practice ran smoothly, without bothering the busy partners. She reasoned that employing her family was necessary to achieve this and that she had acted within the authority given to her by the partners. The tribunal found in her favour, and awarded her £20,000 in compensation.

The above example clearly illustrates why the decision making process needs to be established early in the life of the practice, preferably before the partners start working together. A prospective or new partner would benefit from asking to see the protocol in the agreement before signing it. If none exists, this is a good time to suggest compiling one. Some partners debate the partnership agreement for literally years before finalising it, which is in itself diagnostic of trouble ahead. For busy partners, hammering out a practice agreement or shareholders arguing over their respective rights may seem low priority compared to other pressing issues, but an unsigned agreement will leave individual partners and the practice overall at serious risk.

Which operational model works for me?

The partnership model of practice referred to above is not the only one, and the use of limited companies has a place. The box below highlights the salient points of the two models.

Box 1.2 Partnership or limited company		
	Partnerships	Limited companies
Advantages	• Simplicity • Minor legal obligations • Unless an LLP no obligation to publish accounts • Usually more tax efficient than companies	• Limited liability • Company law requirements comprehensively govern conduct of companies and their officers • Ability to separate owners from workers
Disadvantages	• No limited liability • Cannot separate owners from workers • All partners bound by the agreements made by other partners	• Company law requirements comprehensively govern the conduct of companies and their officers • Financial results of the company have to be published at Companies House for any member of the public to access

Whether a practice opts for a partnership or limited company is a matter of choice. Legally, a partnership does not exist as a separate legal entity, meaning that when the partners leave, the partnership ceases to exist. Limited companies are different. A limited company has its own legal identity with a name and a company number. Closing it requires formal termination through either a formal liquidation process or a request to the Registrar of Companies to strike it off the register. Accordingly, many fledgling businesses start off as partnerships and transfer into limited companies as they evolve. This may be because the business expands and the key individuals involved want the protection of limited liability or because the business has expanded to such a point that it requires funding from external shareholders, for example, the business may become a public company. Company law and tax law

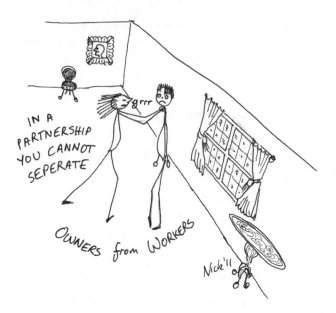

facilitate this healthy development by, for example, allowing business assets to be transferred from a partnership to a company, but the same does not apply in reverse. Starting with a company and moving into a partnership can be done, but the legal and tax framework in the United Kingdom does not make this as easy.

What constitutes practice staff?

In general practice, 'staff' encompasses the entire multidisciplinary team required to deliver a service to patients. The position of staff immediately associated with the practice, such as the receptionists, nurses and partners, is relatively straightforward. Third party associations including consultants and other outsourced clinical and administrative services may be less directly within the GP's control, but will still be viewed by patients as an extension of the practice and integral to the care from their GP. For many businesses, controlling third parties drives managers to despair, as they see their clients, in a GP's case their patients, let down by someone or something beyond their control.

Pre-empting and dealing with this is not straightforward for any business, which explains why so many GPs send their patients to preferred third parties. In business, relationships and trust are recognised as extremely important for success. While GPs may be less conscious of their benefits, the

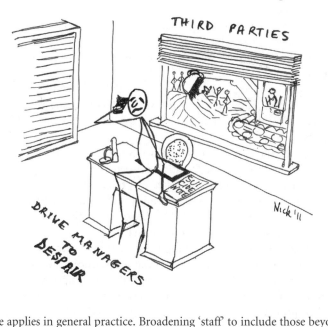

same applies in general practice. Broadening 'staff' to include those beyond the confines of the practice walls or immediate payroll makes routine business activity such as networking, attending meetings and conferences and obtaining feedback from patients less of an anomaly and more a necessity for a healthy practice.

Staff costs are a significant fixed outgoing for any practice, meaning it is worth reviewing the balance and number of staff at regular, ideally annual, intervals to ensure they are still appropriate.

Staff retention and recruitment are also key issues for every business. Staff turnover varies depending on a number of factors, including the nature, location and philosophy of the business. In competitive environments, businesses benchmark their staff turnover figures against those of their competitors. If turnover is higher than the industry norm, they may introduce changes to bring it down. Although it could be argued that general practice is different, the principles still apply. If a practice experiences a high level of staff turnover, it may be worth reviewing its staff policies.

What is great service?

Most successful business sell something, be it cars, corn or advice. The medical profession is no different in this respect which is why everyone inside and outside the practice needs to clearly understand the services it offers. This service must be robust, stand up to scrutiny and criticism and be protected by the partners with the same parental ferocity they would show their children.

To many practices, like many businesses, the range and level of service comprise its unique selling point, or USP. Whether from the partners, other medical staff or the receptionist, this service is key to attracting and keeping patients.

Businesses and practices evolve, and in its early life a new practice may target patients on another GP's list. Dissatisfied patients or those who perceive that the new surgery offers something 'better' may be tempted to move. When this happens in sufficient numbers, the existing practice will experience a 'double whammy' in business terms, in that it will become weaker while at the same time the 'opposition' will become more established.

Business is also dynamic, and the process may be repeated years later when a new group of GPs targets the now established practice. How successful the partners are at defending themselves against the young upstarts will depend on how good they have been at maintaining a sufficiently high level of service for their patients.

Premises: to rent or buy?

A practice takes many forms, from a room in a GP's home to a multilayered purpose built premises. GPs often say they would rather rent than own their premises because of the risks of taking a loan to purchase and develop the site. However, it is fundamentally flawed to assume that renting is less risky than owning.

Taking out a loan carries obvious risks, for example if the partners or business defaults the mortgage company can sue for repayment and ultimately bankrupt the individuals or liquidate the company. Only exceptionally wealthy partners or businesses can purchase premises outright without a loan.

The risks associated with renting may be less obvious but are just as significant. Renting in almost all circumstances requires a lease which sets out the terms between the tenant and the landlord. Two of the most important elements of the lease are the term of the lease with possible break clauses, and the obligation to return the property at the end of the lease to the landlord in the same condition as at the beginning. A developer, who may well become the landlord, will want a secure return on investment. Twenty-five year leases are common in the public–private interface and mean the tenant is obliged to pay rent to the landlord for 25 years. Some leases have break clauses at specific intervals, commonly every five years, when either party can terminate the arrangement. However, many leases recently issued under the Private Finance Initiative (PFI) have no such break clauses.

The fact that the practice is a limited company will not guarantee protection with limited liability status as the landlord will almost certainly require personal guarantees from the GPs who make up the partnership. A lease is an obligation to pay rent. Failure or refusal to do so will result in the landlord suing the tenant for the rent for the rest of the lease. This could happen if for example a practice lost its NHS contract. If the tenant is unable to use the premises or to generate sufficient income to pay the rent, they are left with three main options:

1 Hand the lease back, but only if the landlord is willing to take it back.
2 Sublet the premises, but only if the lease permits this and a new tenant can be found.
3 Refuse to pay with the risk that the landlord will sue and potentially bankrupt the tenant.

Box 1.3 Pros and cons of renting or buying

	Pros	Cons
Rental	• No capital outlay. • Income and expenses should be neutral. • New partners do not need to find capital.	• Obligation to pay rent in future. • Possible dilapidations at end of lease. • Landlord will be entitled to payment even if practice ceases to exist.
Buying	• Possible capital profit. • Ownership gives control. • No need to deal with landlord (e.g. for dilapidations or service charges).	• Requires large loan at outset. • Vulnerable to increases in interest rates. • Problem of raising capital to buy out owners or to buy in.

Failing to appreciate the significance of a lease can catch out the partnership or an individual GP:

Dr John left the Red practice to join a new surgery. Four years later he received a letter from the landlord advising him that, since no rent had been paid on the Red practice for the last six months, he was pursuing Dr John and all his ex-partners for the arrears. Despite Dr John's departure years earlier, he had not been removed from the lease and was still responsible for the rent until it came to an end. Dr John ended up paying £60,000 to the landlord to extract himself from this predicament.

Rent is not the only expense of a lease. Most leases require that the building is returned in the same condition as when the agreement was signed. If the building was new or had been refurbished, considerable funds will be required to maintain it to this standard.

During the term of their 25 year lease, the Purple practice changed the config-uration of their rooms and reception to make them more patient friendly. At the end of the lease they were given a £250,000 dilapidations charge by the landlord to move the rooms back into their original positions.

In order to avoid this charge, the partners had to renegotiate taking on a new lease for a further 25 years. Clearly these negotiations were conducted from a position of weakness as the partners not only had the charge hanging over them but also were unable to argue that they would find alternative, less expensive premises.

To rent or buy . . . that is the question

In many cases, tenants fail to spend sufficient amounts on the property during the term of the lease which results in a large dilapidations charge from the landlord at the end. The partners need to find sufficient money to spend on the property and ensure that all the tenants who have had the benefit of the lease pay their share of the dilapidations if they leave the practice before the end. If the tenants do not make sufficient provision during the term of the lease, then those who are using the property at the end will pay all the refurbishment costs. Recovering a share of costs from former partners who have since retired or died is often impossible. As with saving for tax, the partnership accountant should set aside a dilapidation fund during the term of the lease. This can involve considerable guesswork, and it is better to be prudent than bullish. Businesses faced with a dilapidations bill will obtain estimates from a number of independent contractors, just as one would for building work at home, and negotiate with the landlord before agreeing on a final settlement. Even if sufficient funds have been set aside, this is still good practice.

Renting is not automatically safer than buying, and in the end the partnership will make the decision based on merit. If the partners purchase their premises, then the GPs may need a mortgage, but if they run into trouble they can sell the property, sub-let it to pay the mortgage or find an alternative use for it. If the same GP partnership rents their property and runs into problems, the landlord will force them to continue to pay the rent.

The tax position on either renting or buying is broadly similar. Notional rent income is taxable income. Rent payments for landlords and interest payments for owner-occupiers are both tax deductible expenses. If an owner makes a profit on the sale of their share of the building, that gain is subject to capital gains tax (CGT). Traditionally, there has been a preferential rate of CGT for business assets, including surgery premises. This was called retirement relief, then business taper relief, and it is now labelled as entrepreneur relief. This preferential rate can be lost by accounting for the rent and interest in a way which allows HMRC to argue the premises were not a business asset but an investment. This means it is worth taking professional advice to make sure partners keep the preferential rate.

A surgery building will normally carry two values. The first value is that for the bricks and mortar of the building, and the second is based on the generated rental. The following case shows why it is so important to plan for negative equity:

The Orange practice was given the opportunity to purchase its health centre. The building was not ideal, but the GPs there had been increasingly fed up with poor maintenance and inexplicable but expensive charges. After seeking professional advice, the PCT set the notional rent at £48,000. Using this figure together with an assumed current market investment return of 6%, the capital value was set at £800,000,that is, £800,000 × 6% = £48,000. In fact, the building was valued at £500,000. The PCT value stood up in the light of the proposed rental, but the GPs were all in their early 50s and needed to consider what would happen on their retirement. If the practice were disbanded or if the PCT decided to move it out of the building, they would be left with negative equity. Younger GPs might have taken the risk, but in this case the partners decided not to proceed.

Appealing to your patients

In business, patients correspond to clients, target audiences or purchasers. Whatever the term used, they are essentially the end users of the product on offer and they usually pay to receive it. Alternatively, sufficient numbers use the product to attract third parties such as advertisers, in which case the end user attracts money indirectly. Businesses compete with each other to attract and keep end users, and they view marketing as an essential part of their activity. Most successful businesses have a separate marketing budget, which is so important that it is ring-fenced, this means whatever the general trading conditions, the marketing spend remains protected. GPs as a rule take a conservative attitude to marketing and active competition. Having said that, if a practice exists, whether it likes it or not, it is necessarily in competition at some level. Professional etiquette and distaste at poaching patients from fellow GPs are of course a consideration, but money has always followed patients in UK general practice. This means a practice offering a superior service which patients want to take advantage of will generate financial reward.

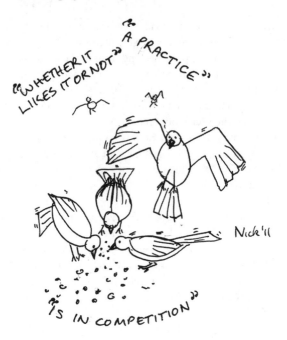

Key points

- Every practice needs a healthy cash flow to survive.
- Profitability is the measure of the practice's ability to earn money.
- Solvency is the state of a practice's financial wealth at any one time.
- A partnership is not the only model in general practice.
- A practice needs concerted direction to achieve its goals.
- 'Staff' extend beyond the practice walls and the payroll.
- Agree which decisions should be made on an individual, majority or unanimous basis.
- Do not assume that leasing premises is a lower risk than buying.
- Plan carefully to ensure that the maximum CGT relief is obtained on sale of business assets.
- A practice offering superior services will generate higher financial rewards.

Chapter 2 **The challenge that is staff**

Staff management is complex, which is why there are thousands of books on the subject and a range of methods in operation in large and small businesses around the world. For these reasons the authors have not attempted to write a definitive guide for GPs, but rather to give them broad principles to consider together with parallels in business which partners can draw on and adapt if they wish.

'You're fired!'

The days of 'trial by sherry' for practice staff are long over. Employment law and European legislation alone make it vital for every employer to understand the complexities and pitfalls of employing and managing staff today. Most commercial organisations have either highly skilled human resources departments or at least access to HR expertise through consultants. Many businesses send their senior managers on regular update courses on employment law and key management issues.

Unfortunately most GPs have had little or no training in staff recruitment, retention and management. They often rely on gut instinct or trial and error, believing that because they can manage patients they can manage staff. Many delegate the responsibility to the practice manager. Delegation is fine, but it can have serious pitfalls if you know less about the issues involved than the person you have hired to act on your behalf.

Commercial organisations do not invest in staff training for altruistic reasons but because it pays them to do so. The costs of expensive litigation are significant, but it is the hidden costs including the time taken, the sheer stress on the partners concerned and the deleterious effect on staff morale which often debilitate a practice. GPs are now fully aware of the stresses involved in patient litigation but staff litigation is just as damaging.

How to Manage Your GP Practice, First Edition. Farine Clarke and Laurence Slavin.
© 2012 John Wiley & Sons, Ltd. Published 2012 by John Wiley & Sons, Ltd.

Employment law is one of those key areas where employers 'do not know what they do not know'. By this we mean the ignorance surrounding employment law is so great that it is only when the employer finds themselves in a tribunal they realise how little they knew about what went wrong. The need to follow correct procedures and processes when recruiting, managing and dismissing staff cannot be emphasised enough. Therefore, whatever the size of your practice, it is worth ensuring that at least one partner or director and one key staff member attend a legal update course at least once every two years. In turn, they can update other senior members of the team.

Do what's right for the practice

Almost every business needs staff, and almost everyone in business knows that staff take up time and resources. The balance between ensuring your staff aid the business without being a drain on it is a fine one and a key to success.

'Do what's right for the patient' is a familiar mantra for GPs which helps to guide them through complex decision making processes. 'Do what's right for the practice' is an equally important but less well recognised mantra when it comes to staff management. If partners put the interests of the practice first in all decisions, it will help them in the most difficult aspects of running a successful team, namely managing staff underperformance, discipline and redundancy. If partners always prioritise the practice, all their decisions will be consistent and objective. This means two GPs from the same practice will be far less likely to give two differing decisions. In turn, staff will understand the collective position of the partners leaving no room for a divide and rule culture. In the long term this will protect the interests of staff as well.

Practices differ in the number and type of staff they require. Having said that, the typical practice will spend one third of its turnover, or income, on staff, one third on overheads, leaving one third as profits for the partners. GPs in common with other small business owners can be inappropriately defensive about their staff costs, not least out of loyalty to their employees.

A three-partner practice with turnover of £560,000 spending 50% of its income on staff is overspending by more than £95,000 compared to its peers. It would be negligent not to investigate the reasons for this extra spend, but these are often complex and may be emotional as well as practical:

The Purple practice spent more than 50% of its income on staff. The practice manager was defensive about staffing levels and tended to compensate for her own weaknesses by employing another assistant. In turn, and symptomatic of the root of the problem, the partners were reluctant to deal with the issue. When the accountant visited he noticed a fully manned reception area with chatting staff and a queue of waiting patients. He tentatively suggested that the staffing levels might be too high, not least because of the salary bill. The partners responded with, 'Well, we hear what you say, but it feels all right to us'.

The Purple practice's response to their accountant ignores the evidence, but it is surprisingly common amongst those running small businesses. This is a classic example of avoiding confronting the issue and instead doing what 'feels right'. What feels right may be what feels most comfortable, but it is wrong for the practice and ultimately damaging to the business and the partners.

Recruitment is now a minefield

Legislation governing recruitment, whether in a small business or a large commercial organisation, is now well established and ignoring the rules is no longer an option for any employer. Discrimination, be it by age, sex or ethnic origin, has clearly never been acceptable but today even those employers who do not intentionally discriminate can find themselves accused of doing so. For this reason it is vital to understand employment law at every stage, from the moment a practice advertises a post, through the selection process, to levels of staff pay, and finally management itself. As with patient litigation, staff today are far more aware of their rights, and quicker to sue employers than they were even ten years ago. Sadly a ruthless few view this as a legitimate way to extract money from employers. While trust and instinct are still valuable assets in the employer-employee relationship, the only way to genuinely protect a practice is to put the correct processes in place and be fully aware of the issues involves.

As an illustration of how things have changed, consider the following innocent ad placed by a GP practice for a receptionist:

Dynamic, energetic, dedicated receptionist required for busy practice. Must be good with people, have excellent communication skills, and be flexible about timings as appointments can overrun at end of the day.

This seemingly harmless advertisement immediately conjures an image of what is required. Yet a potential applicant who is over aged 50 could accuse the practice of age discrimination, claiming 'dynamic and energetic' are biased towards youth. A non-native Caucasian might say that 'excellent communication skills' rules out those with a less than perfect command of English or a strong accent, and is therefore racially discriminatory. A mother with children may protest that 'flexibility' at the end of the day is tantamount to sexual discrimination. How can a woman who needs to be with her family be at the surgery when she should be at home?

At the other end of the spectrum, an increasing number of employers are being sued by people they have not even hired. In actions reminiscent of ambulance chasing in the United States, there are unscrupulous individuals who apply for jobs, and sue potential employers after failing to be either short-listed or hired. The grounds for complaint are often some technicality in the advertisement, or an unfair and biased selection process at interview. This may seem extreme, but just as patient litigation began slowly decades ago, the tide of staff litigation is upon us and will sadly only increase with time.

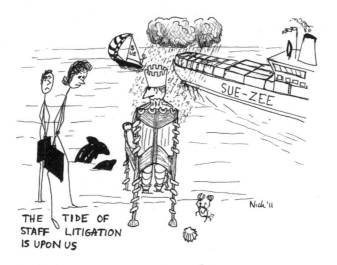

THE TIDE OF STAFF LITIGATION IS UPON US

There are numerous guidelines on how to advertise positions today and GPs would do well to familiarise themselves with these. If in doubt it is worth consulting a professional body or a legal expert before placing a recruitment advertisement. As a general principle, all advertisements should be:
1   Able to withstand scrutiny were they ever presented in a tribunal.
2   Nondiscriminatory in every sense. This means avoid terms which could be construed to favour a particular age, ethnic group or sex.
One might think that this will result in rather flat, boring advertisements, and that may well be true. However, in light of the threat of litigation, it is far better to be cautious than gung ho.

I like you … you remind me of me

There is always a danger of recruiting individuals who have similar characteristics to one's own. Like-minded people gravitate towards each other, as do those with similar educational experiences or those from common backgrounds. This is also true when it comes to promotion. In business this tendency to hire and promote those who are familiar is very well recognised and known as the 'mini me' phenomenon. While it is important to be able to work within cohesive teams, the danger of the mini me is that the make up of staff will be too similar leaving gaps in expertise. Furthermore faults will be replicated rather than corrected. This was the case in the Black practice.

Good HR consultants are geared towards achieving a balanced skill set, particularly in small teams, but they can be expensive and GPs rarely use them. As the demands and expertise of practices change partners may find it increasingly cost- effective and useful to access third-party HR advice.

In the meantime the recruitment procedure outlined below, which is used in business, highlights the need for built-in legal protection as well as methods to avoid the mini me phenomenon within the practice.

Selection of candidates for interview

Before calling candidates for interview, compile a clear, written, job description, together with a list of attributes or qualifications the practice requires from the prospective employee. CVs or written applications can then be checked against these lists and scored accordingly. This means if a potential employee ever queries why they were not selected for interview, the practice can clearly demonstrate that their CV did not score sufficiently well compared with those of other applicants. Practices by their nature are part of the community, meaning staff are often local and known to the partners. Scoring CVs in this way also protects partners from bias at the outset. They cannot be accused of hiring an individual because they are a 'friend' or neighbour.

The interview process

Conduct interviews with at least two staff members in the room, as just one will lay the practice open to claims of discrimination or bias.

The interviewers should work through an agreed list of question to give the interview structure and make sure every applicant is given the same opportunity to shine and is scored fairly against each question. Of course the interview can be peppered with general conversation to keep it relaxed and human, but interviewing is a vigorous process and the practice must be able to demonstrate that it conducted a fair and thorough procedure at all times.

Once the interviews are completed and the scores totalled, the candidate with the highest mark should, technically, be offered the job. If the practice is sued, it can clearly demonstrate that it followed a fair and thorough procedure. Following this process may result in selecting the person whom

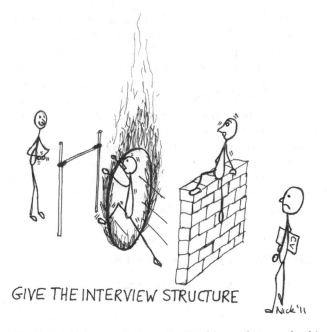

GIVE THE INTERVIEW STRUCTURE

is least 'liked', but, if the practice has prioritised its needs correctly, this will also be the best person for the job. GPs will always have a view about personality and fit with other team members and may decide to justify making a different final choice. But if they do then at least this will be an informed, carefully made, decision, which they are able to defend.

Did you write this reference?

References are tricky in many respects. In business an increasing number of companies do not give references other than to say a person worked in the firm from such and such a date, and basically did the job according to its title. In the old days this would have been regarded as a 'bad' reference, but today this is simply standard practice and once again litigation is at its core. An employee who is offered a job pending references and then fails to get it can, and increasingly does, sue their ex-employer for defamation. Having said that it is naïve to imply that the process of calling ex-employers for information 'off the record' does not go on, or that employers don't recommend candidates to each other on an informal basis. They clearly do.

When taking up or giving references, it helps to understand their role in the recruitment process. On a practical level finding out as much as possible

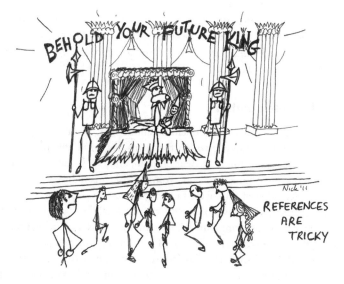

about a prospective candidate beforehand, while clearly useful, can leave one exposed.

The following example illustrates the legal minefield surrounding references:

Paula applied for the job of assistant manager at the Magenta practice. She performed well at interview, showed considerable promise, and was hired. After a few months her work deteriorated so much that the partners reviewed her CV and reference, believing they may have made a mistake when they originally read them. Her documents were all consistent with her appointment. It was only when one of the GPs telephoned her referee that alarm bells started to ring as he was extremely guarded. There then followed a series of probing phone calls, and eventually her referee admitted that Paula's work had deteriorated shortly after employment in her previous practice in an identical manner. During what he considered to be an informal chat, he had suggested she considered leaving, not least because she seemed unhappy. Paula had left but then sued his practice for constructive dismissal. She won an out of court settlement together with an assurance that the episode would not be discussed in future references. She won because the correct disciplinary procedure had not been followed and also because an employer who suggests that 'things are not working out' or they should 'consider leaving' can be accused of making it impossible for an employee to stay in their job. This is the basis for a constructive dismissal claim. It emerged that Paula was a professional litigant and had been through this process several times. On each occasion she had extracted a compensation payment from a naïve employer. This time the GPs were armed with the right information and followed correct procedure to performance-manage Paula out of her job.

In my humble opinion ...

Former employers often face a dilemma about what to say to prospective employers about a candidate whom they consider unsuitable for the post: should they be totally honest in their opinion, and risk litigation, or should they remain silent about their concerns and risk misleading the new employer? Advice between employers, but not between lawyers, varies according to individual levels of bravado, but the correct legal approach is to simply state the facts without giving a subjective opinion. This is not as unsatisfactory as it might seem because employees who do 'badly' in one place can do extremely well in another. The reasons are often multifactorial and relate to the differences in personalities, ethos, training, support networks and mentors between different work places. Ex-employers frequently have little or no insight into the significance of these differences.

You do the management ... I'll get on with the real work

Many GPs deride the term *management* even more than *money* in the professional context. To them management is a nebulous, time consuming specialty, which surrounds itself in jargon to justify its existence and invariable involves an extraordinary amount of paperwork and procedure. Worst of all, management and those who are exercised by it combine to detract GPs from the job in hand, namely to care for patients. If GPs had wanted to be managers they would have done MBAs not become doctors. Furthermore because they deal with the complexities of patient care on a daily basis they consider themselves more than capable of managing staff.

It is of course absolutely true that many GP skills are transferable and family doctors do have an instinctive understanding of what motivates and helps their patients.

However, staff management is not the same as patient management and the relationship between GPs and their staff is very different from the doctor-patient dynamic. One major difference is that staff in a practice function within a team and are frequently motivated and demotivated as a team. Factors affecting one staff member will have a knock-on effect on colleagues with a resultant impact on the practice as a whole.

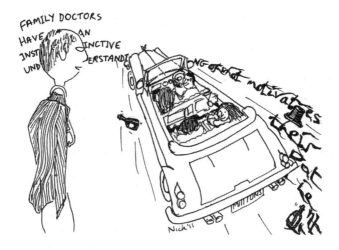

Unlike patients who view their care as confidential, staff will often discuss sensitive practice matters freely with each other. Consider how many times a conversation in your practice has started with the words 'Don't tell anyone but ...' before the rumour is circulated throughout the building? This is not the same as discussing patient details which are clearly governed by confidentiality rules and which staff understand are an intrinsic requirement of their job. Personal matters surrounding pay, promotion, discipline and health are frequently treated with less discretion and discussed internally before the partners have made any formal statements.

Similarly the GP-patient power gradient is widely different from that between GPs and their staff. As a rule patients respect their doctor for knowing more about medicine than they do. In the outside world everyone has a view on what constitutes good management and the country is full of staff who feel that their bosses are 'useless' managers. This view is by no means unique to general practice, but the lack of formal management training and human resources support leaves GPs more exposed to criticism.

GPs do not need to 'learn' management for the sake of it and being good managers will not necessarily make them better doctors. The reason for GPs to familiarise themselves with, and employ, management techniques is for their own benefit. Doing so ensures their practice runs smoothly, is protected from undue tensions and litigation and is ultimately more successful. Good management is associated with a content, productive workforce while poor practice results in a demotivated, less effective one.

How a practice deals with its staff as a whole is up to the individual partners, but the process is an active rather than passive one which means it is helpful to be up to date with management tools and techniques.

Ensure the staff handbook is up-to-date

There are several examples of best management practice but one of the overriding principles is to ensure the correct processes are in place. As a general rule, all staff should have:

1 A written job description explaining the role and responsibilities. This is reviewed on joining so that any issues can be aired and resolved at the outset. How detailed or rigid the job description is will vary according to the role and practice philosophy. Disputes frequently arise over what is, or is not, included in this document making it a useful reference point.

2 An annual appraisal with the direct line manager. In this meeting the good and less satisfactory parts of the job are discussed openly, without distraction. At the end of the appraisal an action plan for the following year is agreed between both parties. This plan is akin to a contract for the way ahead and focuses on those issues of concern together with constructive ways to improve performance on both sides. For many employees this is the only opportunity to talk frankly with their managers in a structured manner, and for many managers this is the only opportunity to ring fence time for a constructive review with the employee. The mere action of having an appraisal makes staff feel they are being treated professionally and taken seriously in their job. This in itself improves job satisfaction and performance.

3 An annual salary review: most businesses now conduct these separately from the appraisal because it can be confusing to say tell someone they are doing wonderfully well in their job but they are not getting a pay increase. Several factors will influence rates of pay in a business and these will be independent of how well someone is performing in a role for which they are already paid.

4 All practices need a staff handbook which is circulated to every new employee on joining. This serves three functions: it reassures the joiner that the practice is run professionally, it acts as a reference book to deal with work related queries and it sets the employment standards within the practice. The handbook gives as much detail as possible about the practice, its approach to staff and what is expected in return. All the processes, including staff remuneration, maternity pay, sickness, complaints and disciplinary procedures, are detailed in the handbook. There is considerable reference material for staff handbooks available. A senior member of the practice team should be responsible for reviewing and revising the handbook on an annual basis.

Guess what motivates me?

To say that remuneration is the key to staff retention is a myth. Adequate remuneration is important because it confirms a value for a particular skill or job. In turn a perceived shortfall in salary may be one reason why employers look around for a new position, but it is rarely the sole consideration. A new job which clearly offers promotion, provides new opportunities or meets a practical need such as a shorter journey time to work will always be attractive to staff. But most staff do not resign for monetary reasons alone. Far more leave because they 'were not appreciated'. This does not mean that you, as the employer, were obliged to appreciate them, but it may matter to partners who find themselves losing staff they would rather have kept.

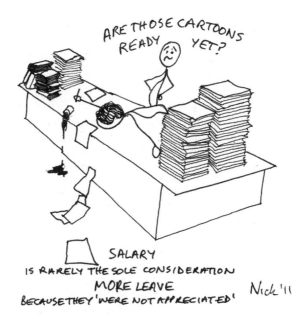

I told you I was unhappy

The key to staff retention is job satisfaction. Individuals may believe they are slightly under-paid but if at the same time they know they are making a valid contribution and are appreciated they accept this. Making a person feel appreciated is in itself a challenge. GPs are very hard taskmasters when it comes to themselves, which is understandable considering their training and the nature of their profession. Being self-critical can also mean that they are equally hard on their staff, believing that if no one is dying then everyone should just get on with it. This approach although not unheard of in business is rarer and not quite so engrained in the psyche of many businessmen and women. Their life experiences are closer to that of their staff in many aspects and are a far cry from the harsh realities of life and death which doctors deal with on a daily basis.

Rewarding staff rewards the practice

Commercial organisations commonly set target-driven bonuses to motivate staff and increase profits. While this remains rare in general practice some business minded practices have found it a useful tool.

Box 2.1 Examples of good and bad targets for staff		
Good	Bad	Reason
Based on increasing specific source of Income		Staff can directly influence this income source
	Based on increasing overall profits	Profits affected by decisions by others apart from staff
Based on reducing specific expense		Staff can directly influence this expense
	Based on increasing solvency	Solvency affected by decisions by others apart from staff

Rewarding staff well can in turn reap long-term benefits for the practice. As with most messages to staff rewards are better given on a consistent basis rather than as one-off grand gestures. Surprises are fun and can improve staff morale, but they should still be part of an overall plan.

Rewards take many forms ranging from individual bonuses which can be financial or other to team bonuses such as staff trips together. Some practices take expert coordinators on away-days to give structure and more tangible benefit. A typical away-day or weekend will involve a series of team building sessions, followed by a relaxing informal dinner possibly with a motivational or humorous guest speaker. This approach is common to many businesses and while they can sometimes appear either manufactured or expensive, they invariably benefit both individual employees and the team overall.

Being rewarded is a bonus

Businesses frequently reward their staff with straightforward financial bonuses which are set against specific targets. The targets may be a combination of personal targets, such as those specific to the member of staff and over which they will have direct control, and group or team targets which are set against the wider aims of the business. While the individual has less control over these he or she can still contribute to them. Some businesses set bonuses against targets over which the individual has no control or input, believing that if the business does well everyone will benefit and vice versa. The range and type of target will depend on the business and while this practice is less common in medicine it can be adapted for GP staff. It is up to partners to decide firstly if they wish to target staff on principle and secondly what form targets should take.

Practice meetings add value

GPs work in greater isolation from their staff compared to other professionals, not least because of the confidential environment needed for the doctor-patient relationship. As a result staff can feel unsupported while the GPs are absent or busy in their consulting rooms. Similarly partners are less aware of day to day nuances within the practice from the dramas with disgruntled patients in the waiting room to the gossip round the coffee machine. If partners can make staff believe they understand the issues they face, they will mitigate against their disruptive effect on the practice. Holding meetings is an activity in itself and while many will argue that there are too many in primary care, regular, structured meetings are excellent for maintaining communication throughout the practice. The net result is the practice will run more efficiently and waste less time A monthly immovable meeting set in everyone's diary is a useful discipline. The day, agenda, chair and list of attendees can all be agreed by individual partners.

One reason managers dislike meeting staff is because they can turn into 'moaning' sessions. Feedback always seems like a good idea until it is given at which point it becomes a list of painful gripes. Constructive staff feedback is more rewarding. A practice policy whereby staff can only bring a problem to the meeting if they also bring two suggested solutions prevents them 'dumping' issues at the GPs feet while at the same time encourages them to actively improve the practice. Not all suggestions have to be adopted immediately but agreeing to one or two strengthens the relationship between partners and staff and makes employees feel they can impact their work environment.

Property isn't the only thing worth stealing

Theft in the business environment is not confined to obvious targets such as money, stationery, computers and even toilet paper. Assets such as time and information or data are less tangible but highly valuable targets.

In addition to all of these, GP surgeries also play host to even more dangerous items like prescription pads and drugs:

During the annual accounts review, Dr Cohen, the senior partner at the Navy practice is Durham, explained they were having difficulties with their new practice manager. The accountant immediately recognised his name from two different practices on his client list. He had been dismissed from the first for underperforming, coupled with violent mood swings, and from the second, for stealing prescriptions for his own use. At that stage he had had admitted an addiction to prescription drugs.

The partners had felt their practice manager needed help and encouragement rather than to lose another job and Dr Cohen had delegated an afternoon a week to counsel him. In the meantime other members of staff had become increasingly uncomfortable because they found him intimidating and were threatening to leave.

This example illustrates that a surgery is an attractive place for those with a vested interest in being among drugs and doctors.

It also demonstrates that, while helping a member of staff in difficulty is laudable, it is not necessarily in the best interests of the practice and the staff. Even if the partner concerned is an expert in drug rehabilitation he has made his employee his patient and compromised everyone's position. Consider attempting to discipline a staff member you are also treating for drug addiction. Whether or not the approach is ethical it will have an inevitable negative effect on the other partners and the rest of the team, particularly as the practice manager role is such a senior one.

This is an ethical dilemma, but had the GPs done what was best for the practice first, and dealt with the performance issue, they may well have dismissed the new manager but at least his drug addiction would have come to light and he could have received the right treatment openly and professionally by a third party.

Should I treat you or pay you?

The above is an extreme example of what can happen when GPs treat their own staff. Doctors are often tempted to do so, even when staff are registered elsewhere, because they consider it helpful, sympathetic and frequently more practical. It can appear disingenuous to refuse to advise someone who is in the same building and clearly needs help, but taking on a dual role is risky and not always in the best interests of the employee, let alone the partner. When boundaries become blurred and the relationship confused both parties are open to abuse. In business there is never a corresponding situation whereby a boss can medically treat an employee. If they could it would not only be considered unethical, but there would also be checks and balances in place and a plethora of policy documents and courses on the subject!

'Me time'

Time deserves special mention as a valuable commodity which is frequently stolen from GPs. Patients, staff and even the soon to be abolished PCT reports all vie for a GP's time, making protecting this a priority. Allocating sufficient time resource to important activities including financial meetings, reading reports and attending conferences, is vital for success. Commercial organisations routinely ring-fence time for work which at first sight may not directly impact the company, because they know that in the long term it will. By contrast, doctors and their staff can hold the misguided view that anything which does not directly involve patients is not proper work. Therefore it is

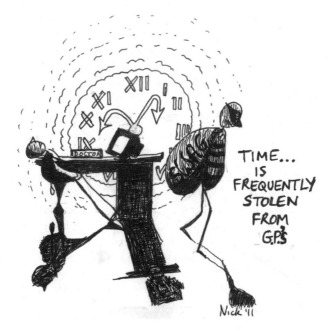

TIME...
IS
FREQUENTLY
STOLEN
FROM
G.P.'s

vital for a successful practice to ensure partners are allocated sufficient, sacrosanct, time for personal and professional development and they should neither feel, nor be made to feel, guilty for doing so.

Discipline: a thorny problem

Disciplining staff is one of the most difficult functions GPs have to exercise as guardians of the practice. The relationship between doctors and their staff is a close bond which has often been strengthened by years of unique, shared experiences, and is based on trust.

Furthermore, the practice is part of the community and many GPs have known not only their staff but also the immediate and extended family sometimes for generations. If this can influence them when it comes to hiring, it definitely comes to mind where discipline and possibly firing are concerned.

This is one reason why the mantra: always put the practice first, was never more relevant than when it comes to discipline. Putting the practice first means it will be obvious to partners when the time has come to start disciplinary procedures and how far to take them. Putting the practice first also means that at all times GPs will think of their staff as a team that needs to function at an optimal level. If one member of the team underperforms, and this is allowed to continue, then all staff will be affected. Similarly staff will look to the partners for consistency; if everyone knows where they stand and is treated the same when boundaries are crossed or rules are broken, then the practice will function smoothly. Inconsistency and favouritism are rightly perceived by staff as unfair and are often at the root of their discontent.

Putting the practice first and being consistent will help partners identify when to act with all practice staff, even when their behaviour is not obviously dramatic or damaging:

Basil joined the successful, motivational Graphite practice in East Anglia as a salaried GP. He was a little slow but produced good quality work and was liked by patients. However, he was short tempered with staff and consistently criticised their work without ever giving positive feedback. One in three complaints by the practice employees was about Basil. Within three months of his appointment, a negative attitude had spread through the team and the staff were generally 'down'. In turn this attitude became tangible to patients. The partners carefully raised the issue with Basil, but he failed to acknowledge that there was a problem so they proceeded to manage him out of the practice. When he left, the whole team cheered up as if a cloud had been lifted.

UNDERPERFORMANCE

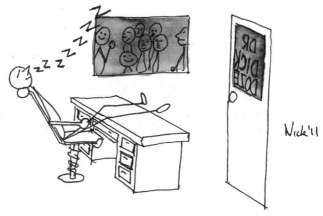

Nick'll

A CONSISTENT & DAMAGING PROBLEM

Disciplinary procedures can save a practice

All practices need a formal disciplinary procedure which is documented in the staff handbook and familiar to the partners and practice manager. It may seem obvious, but all surgeries need to also follow their procedure, partly because this is best practice but also because tribunals invariably find in favour of a complainant whose employers have failed to adhere to a correct disciplinary process. This may seem like a technicality but ignoring it will cost a practice dearly.

Throughout the day managers will steer staff in the right direction, correct mistakes and make suggestions for improvement. All of this is done on an informal basis, is clearly good practice and the majority of staff respond positively.

When there is a serious matter or when underperformance becomes a consistent and damaging problem, managers may decide to formalise the process to demonstrate the gravity of the situation and to try to solve it. At this stage the formal disciplinary procedure kicks in.

The exact formal disciplinary processes will vary between businesses and in larger companies is a HR function. The key stages in a typical procedure for GPs are outlined below.

1   Schedule a meeting between the employee and their direct manager who is often the practice manager, and another representative from the practice.

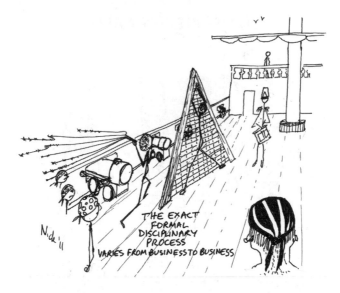

THE EXACT FORMAL DISCIPLINARY PROCESS VARIES FROM BUSINESS TO BUSINESS

Avoid involving a senior member of staff to whom the employee may appeal at a later stage in the process.

2 At the meeting explain this is a disciplinary meeting and state the reasons clearly. Explain the process. Go through the areas of underperformance and explain which areas you wish to improve and how this improvement will be measured. Give a time scale for doing so. Allow the employee to feedback, as they may give credible reasons for the problem which deserve a hearing. Take full and detailed notes of the meeting.

3 Before the time for improvement is over, schedule another meeting to discuss progress. Often the matter will have been resolved by this stage and the procedure although now documented, can be halted. If it is not, express concerns that things are not better. Again allow the member of staff to give reasons. Again take full notes.

4 If there has been no significant improvement by the next meeting issue and record a 'verbal warning' and give a timescale for improvement.

5 If there is no improvement within this time, issue a written warning with a time scale for dismissal.

6 The employee may appeal against the decision at any stage. The appeal will be to a more senior member of staff (often the senior partner).

7 At this final meeting ensure there is a member of staff present to take notes. The appeal should be heard and the employee's statements noted in writing. After this meeting the appeal can either be upheld or rejected. The employee must be sent written notification of the decision.

8 If the decision is to reject the appeal then the employee can be dismissed. Depending on their contract they can either be dismissed with no further notice period and salary, or may reach an agreement with the partners.

Key points

- Litigation against employers and potential employers in on the rise.
- Ensure your recruitment and selection procedures stand up to scrutiny.
- The candidate you like the most may not be the best person for the job.
- Put best practice staff management systems in place.
- Guard against the 'mini-me' phenomenon when recruiting and promoting staff.
- Staff retention is not solely related to remuneration.
- Staff will discuss personal issues with each other.
- Good management will improve the profitability of the practice.
- Useful meetings are helpful for the practice; useless meetings are infuriating.
- Time is as valuable as money but is stolen far more often.

Chapter 3 **Basic practice accounting**

It can take GP partners up to five years of detailed explanations from their accountant before they fully understand the concepts and ideas demonstrated in the figures. This chapter aims to fast forward that timescale and make the accounts instantly meaningful.

De-mystifying the accounts

Double entry bookkeeping was invented by Luca Pacioli, a Franciscan monk, who used it to compile the monastery accounts in Italy. The basic principle is that every transaction has two effects. For instance, if a business makes a sale, it increases sales and also increases the bank balance. A business placing an order for stationery increases the stationery expenses and also increases the liabilities. When the business eventually pays for the stationery, it reduces the liabilities and also reduces the bank balance. In accounting terms each separate part of each transaction is called either a debit or a credit.

This often mystifies non-accountants, but it is helpful to have an understanding of the process that makes this work.

Accountants have a basic accounting equation that says:

$$\text{Assets} - \text{Liabilities} = \text{Capital}$$

If you are familiar with accounts, you will recognise this as a summary of a balance sheet.

The equation can be simply expanded by taking the statement that capital is increased each year by the profits the practice makes.

So, we can restate the equation as follows:

$$\text{Assets} - \text{Liabilities} = \text{Capital from last year} + \text{Profit}$$

How to Manage Your GP Practice, First Edition. Farine Clarke and Laurence Slavin.
© 2012 John Wiley & Sons, Ltd. Published 2012 by John Wiley & Sons, Ltd.

Remember that profit is the difference between income and expenses, so the equation can be developed further:

Assets − Liabilities = Capital from last year + Income − Expenses

Moving the negative items across to make them positive gives the equation:

Assets + Expenses = Capital from last year + Income + Liabilities

This is the equation that underpins every set of accounts, and that deals with both sides of every transaction.

The following examples illustrate the point:

- Transaction 1: Staff costs of £10,000 are paid from the practice bank account. The effect is to increase the expenses and reduce the bank balance (an asset).
- Transaction 2: Fees of £20,000 are paid to the practice bank account. The effect is to increase income and increase the bank account (an asset).
- Transaction 3: Stationery costing £2,000 is bought on credit. The effect is to increase expenses and increase liabilities.
- Transaction 4: The stationery creditor is repaid £750. The bank account (an asset) is reduced and the liability is reduced.

Inserting these four transactions into the equation has the following effect:

	Assets £	+	Expenses £	=	Last years' capital	Income + £	Liabilities + £
Transaction 1	− 10,000		+ 10,000				
Transaction 2	+ 20,000					+ 20,000	
Transaction 3			+ 2,000				+ 2,000
Transaction 4	− 750						− 750
Total	+ 9,250		+ 12,000	=		+ 20,000	+ 1,250

Accountants call this a 'trial balance'. A trial balance which is equal on both sides gives some assurance that all the practice transactions have been properly accounted for, and the accounting process is reliable.

At the Black practice accounts review, the senior partner, Dr Thomas, suggested that the bank balance was understated by £2,000 and asked the accountant to simply raise the figure by this amount. His accountant cautioned that he would need to demonstrate clearly where the £2,000 came from to make the practice accounts balance. There then followed some argument, during which the accountant stressed that it was in the partners' best interests to ensure their accounts did balance. He explained that every single transaction which went through the bank accounts and the petty cash, and even some outside the accounts, required to be stated with its double effects to achieve accurate year-end accounts.

Many GPs have never seen a trial balance, but they will be familiar with the following example, in which the accountants take the trial balance and split it up into two sections:

$$\text{Trial Balance : Assets} + \text{Expenses} = \text{Capital from last year}$$
$$+ \text{Income} + \text{Liabilities}$$

This splits into (1) assets, capital and liabilities; and (2) expenses and income.

The assets, capital and liabilities are put into what is called a 'balance sheet', while the expenses and income are inserted into a 'profit and loss' account.

Using the numbers from this trial balance, the figures appear as follows:

Profit and loss account	
Income	£20,000
Less expenses	− 12,000
Profit	8,000

Balance sheet	
Assets	9,250
Less liabilities	− 1,250
Total	8,000

Opening capital (from last year)	0
Profit (from profit and loss account)	8,000
Total	8,000

From what appeared to be a meaningless statement, the trial balance has generated two vital documents, namely the profit and loss account which explains how profitable the practice has been during the year, and the balance sheet which shows the extent of the assets and liabilities in the practice. In other words, the solvency of the practice.

A set of practice accounts will commonly exceed ten pages, but the profit and loss account and the balance sheet are the two most important ones for GPs to focus on. The rest of the accounts give the detailed explanations and workings which back up these two documents.

Which accounting system is best for your practice?

It is clearly critical that the practice has a bookkeeping system which keeps an accurate record of the day to day transactions and also facilitates the production of the accounts.

Accountants use a number of tools to ensure the accuracy of the accounts of which the bank reconciliation is the most important. In this process, the accountant takes the bank balance at the beginning of the year and adds in all the receipts from the practice accounting records. Next, all the payments from the practice accounting records are deducted. The number left should equal the actual bank balance on the bank statement at the end of the year. If the two figures differ, the accountant has to go through all the year's transactions to find what is missing. This is an arduous task, and can add considerably to the practice's accountancy costs. This is also why the accounting system must not only properly identify every item which goes through the accounts, but also be 100% complete as just one missing item will necessitate the accountant searching through all the entries to find the difference in the bank reconciliation.

It is worth discussing a potential accounting system with the practice accountant to ensure its functionality and compatibility will meet the needs of the practice. As a minimum, the accounting system needs to break down the receipts and payments into assets, liabilities, income and expenses, at the broadest level. As already stated, it must also be 100% complete. Most proprietary accounting software will meet these needs, but if the partners prefer to use a bespoke system they need to be sure it will achieve their aims.

Dr Jones developed his own accounting system and handed his accountant a long computerised list of every receipt and payment made into the practice bank account. He was proud that he had completed his own bank reconciliation which demonstrated that his list started with the opening bank balance and ended with the closing balance. Unfortunately, while the list was clearly complete, it failed to explain or analyse the transactions, and did not break down expenditure on assets, or expenses, or income from receipts. To make the list useful, Dr Jones' accountant had to review every transaction and assign it correctly. Dr Jones was disappointed that he had wasted so much time entering the data, which proved, in the end, to be useless.

There are two types of software on the market. One is the 'accounting' package which manages the double entry effect of each transaction and produces a profit and loss account and balance sheet; examples include Sage and Quickbooks. The other is a 'spreadsheet' package which summarises the accounting entries in a manner that facilitates production of the end of year accounts; examples include Excel and GP Accounts.

The accounting package is not automatically preferable to the spreadsheet, and the choice of system depends on the ability of the person keeping the accounting records rather than the system itself. In double entry accounting every transaction has two financial effects, and the advantage of the accounting package is that the user only has to make one entry and the program will automatically generate the other one. In the bank payment section in Sage, for example, enter an Electricity payment of £1,000 and the program will automatically enter £1,000 of Electricity costs and deduct £1,000 from the bank balance. Difficulties occur when the user makes a mistake: if the £1,000 was mistakenly entered as a Cleaning payment, the journal section of the accounting system would need to be adjusted by increasing cleaning costs by £1,000 and reducing electricity costs by £1,000. In the journal the two entries are manually put into the system, and no automatic double entry works in the journal.

In accounting terms, the adjustment is as follows:

1. Debit Electricity   £1,000
and
2. Credit Cleaning   £1,000

Does double entry mean I go in twice?

Difficulties arise if the user does not fully understand how double entry bookkeeping works and does not know how to make the correction. A feature of accounting programs is that they do not allow you to cancel an entry that has been made. This preserves an "audit trail." So a user who does not understand how double entry bookkeeping works may produce a whole series of transactions, each one not quite achieving its goal and each one turning what should have been a simple entry into a complex series of not quite self-cancelling transactions.

Although companies selling these systems do offer training to new purchasers, double entry cannot be learnt in a week and in reality it takes most accountants about a year to practice it with confidence.

This is why a competent bookkeeper in the practice should be encouraged to use an accounting program and a less competent one actively discouraged and offered a spreadsheet program instead. These operate on a simpler level: the user makes an entry in the appropriate expense column, and the program allocates the figure to a total column. It is relatively easy for the accountant to produce a trial balance, a profit and loss account and a balance sheet from the total column.

The detailed accounts below from the Sunnihill Health Centre are presented to inform readers about the salient elements of the financial documents.

SUNNIHILL HEALTH CENTRE
ACCOUNTS
FOR THE YEAR ENDED
31 MARCH 2010

PRACTICE INFORMATION

PARTNERS: Dr Ghode
                                        Dr Stern
                                        Dr Hart

SURGERY ADDRESS: Health Centre
                                        170 Replay Road
                                        Chichester
                                        West Sussex

ACCOUNTANTS: Davison and Sons
                                        Chartered Accountants
                                        Deer House
                                        8 Lyme Avenue
                                        Midhurst
                                        West Sussex

CLIENT REFERENCE:

**SUNNIHILL HEALTH CENTRE
ACCOUNTS
FOR THE YEAR ENDED
31 MARCH 2010**

CONTENTS

	PAGE
Accountants' Report	1
Partners' Certificate	2
Profit and Loss Account	3
Balance Sheet	4
Schedules of Income	5–7
Notes to the Accounts	8–10

SUNNIHILL HEALTH CENTRE
ACCOUNTS
FOR THE YEAR ENDED
31 MARCH 2010

ACCOUNTANTS' REPORT TO THE PARTNERS
OF HEALTH CENTRE
ON THE UNAUDITED ACCOUNTS

We have compiled the accounts of your practice which comprise a profit and loss account, a balance sheet and related notes from the accounting records and information and explanations given to us.

The accounts are not intended to achieve full compliance with the provisions of UK Generally Accepted Accounting Principles.

Our work has been undertaken so that we might compile the accounts that we have been engaged to compile, report to you that we have done so and state those matters that we have agreed to state to you in this report and for no other purpose. To the fullest extent permitted by law, we do not accept or assume responsibility to anyone other than to you for our work, or for this report.

We have carried out this engagement in accordance with technical guidance issued by the Institute of Chartered Accountants in England & Wales and have complied with the ethical guidance laid down by the Institute.

You have approved the accounts for the year ended 31 March 2010 and have acknowledged your responsibility for them, for the appropriateness of the accounting basis and for providing all information and explanations necessary for their compilation.

We have not verified the accuracy or completeness of the accounting records or information and explanations you have given to us and we do not, therefore, express any opinion on the financial information.

Signed:
Date:

Page 1: The accountants' report

The accountant sets out the terms on which their work has been done. It is straightforward, although it is worth noting that unlike the medical profession and the legal profession, the accountancy profession is open to unqualified individuals to practice without sanction. Typically the accountant will have the letters FCA, ACA, FCCA or ACCA after their name confirming they are a member of a chartered institute and are properly qualified to act as an accountant. Other letters merit investigation. Some represent qualifications that can simply be applied for online with little evidence of ability.

2

SUNNIHILL HEALTH CENTRE
ACCOUNTS
FOR THE YEAR ENDED
31 MARCH 2010

PARTNERS' CERTIFICATE

We certify that, to the best of our knowledge and belief, the accounting records provided, together with the information and explanations given to Davison and Sons, constitute a true and correct record of the transactions of our practice for the year ended 31 March 2010, and we confirm that the accounts have our approval.

....
Dr. Ghode

....
Dr. Stern

....
Dr. Hart

Dated 2010

Page 2: The partners' certificate

The partners confirm that they have approved the accounts as prepared by the partnership accountants. This page is also straightforward, but any partner signing these accounts is confirming that he or she agrees with them. A partner making a subsequent claim having already signed off the accounts dealing with this claim will face difficulties justifying a change. It is therefore preferable for partners to be certain they understand the accounts, even if this means asking seemingly straightforward questions, rather than to simply rubber stamp them with a signature.

Dr Jolly joined Dr Khan's practice. The accounts for their first year together showed Dr Jolly in debt for £20,000. In that year he had only received a limited amount of the practice earnings, while at the same time he was charged the full share of the expenses. Very shortly afterwards, Dr Khan dissolved the practice and asked Dr Jolly to repay the £20,000. Dr Jolly refused, claiming he had been the victim of deceit and did not owe the money. In turn Dr Khan claimed that the monies followed the agreement between them. Both parties appointed legal advisors, but Dr Jolly was advised to pay the £20,000 as he had signed off the accounts, which set out the reasons for his over-drawn element.

**SUNNIHILL HEALTH CENTRE
PROFIT AND LOSS ACCOUNT
FOR THE YEAR ENDED 31 MARCH 2010**

3

	Sch £	2010 £	2009 £	£
Fees Earned (Before deduction of £41,699 Superannuation)	1	568,867		549,097
Reimbursements	2	65,305		44,082
Other Income	3	16,606		12,101
		650,778		605,280

LESS OVERHEADS

Salaries and Wages	173,112	150,652
Note Summarising	6,506	5,270
Salaried Assistant	121,498	68,684
Staff Welfare	3,157	3,701
Staff Pension	6,787	5,784
Staff Training	26	1,140
Locums	26,004	17,863
Deputising and Co-op Service	1,917	1,066
Drugs	17,722	13,643
Telephone	6,557	5,119
Computer Expenses	1,580	6,273
Printing, Postage and Stationery	8,068	6,749
Subscriptions	999	1,719
General Expenses	147	151
Hire of Equipment	516	473
Courses and Conferences	424	(126)
Advertising	869	361
Travelling	184	207
Repairs and Maintenance	2,589	700
Insurance	1,150	969
Rent and Rates	24,480	24,000
Parking Permit Charge	2,315	2,920
Health Centre Charges	(607)	10,782
Levies	3,507	2,782
Bank Interest and Charges	914	239
Legal and Professional Fees	3,612	1,533
Accountancy	4,700	4,477
Depreciation	558	656
	(419,291)	(337,787)
NET PROFIT FOR THE YEAR (NOTE 1)	231,487	267,493

Page 3: The profit and loss account

This key page deals with the profitability of the practice, and represents the difference between the income and expenses. In this case, a simple review of page 3 shows the practice made profits of £231,487. This practice has 2.25 full time equivalent (FTE) partners, so a full time partner's share of profits would be £102,883. The following points are worthy of note:

1 The monies the partners take out of the practice are not shown on this page.

2 Any assets purchased from practice monies are not shown on this page.

3 Income and expenses are included, not as monies are received or paid, but as income is earned and expenses are incurred.

A common question is "How much do I earn as a partner?" The answer is that a partner's earnings are their profit share from the practice. This is also the figure that is used to calculate their tax, not the amount of money that they take out of the practice.

4

SUNNIHILL HEALTH CENTRE
BALANCE SHEET
AS AT 31 MARCH 2010

	Note £	2010 £	2009 £	£
FIXED ASSETS				
Tangible Assets	2		3,162	3,720
CURRENT ASSETS				
Stock of Drugs		2,330		2,330
Sundry Debtors and Prepayments		61,682		63,741
Main Bank Account		37,893		48,902
Building Society Account		1,619		21,855
Cash in Hand		1,350		396
		104,874		137,224
CURRENT LIABILITIES				
Taxation		33,116		38,237
Superannuation		7,414		5,476
Sundry Creditors and Accruals		5,634		17,820
		46,164		61,533
NET CURRENT ASSETS			58,710	75,691
			61,872	79,411
REPRESENTED BY:				
CURRENT ACCOUNTS	3			
Dr. Ghode			25,304	27,580
Dr. Stern			21,856	33,866
Dr. Hart			14,712	17,965
			61,872	79,411

Page 4: The balance sheet

This second key page from the accounts is derived from the trial balance. The balance sheet has two distinct sections, one showing the assets and liabilities in the practice, and the other showing how much of those net assets each partner is entitled to. The accounts above show the practice has net current assets of £58,710 and overall net assets of £61,872. The net current assets are the difference between the current assets and current liabilities. By 'current', we mean they are likely to pass through the bank account in the next 12 months. The term 'net current assets' is also referred to as the 'working capital', and is a vital measure of the solvency of a practice. In this case the net current assets have decreased from £75,691 to £58,710, in other words, there is £16,981 less money than at the beginning of the year. If this was intentional and controlled, it is not a problem, but if the partners were unaware of this, it suggests they were over-drawing (i.e. setting their monthly drawings higher than the profits that were being generated).

It is important to recognise and understand the causes of over-drawing, and adjust them to be in line with the profits. In order to provide some contingency a practice would ideally bring drawings below the profits. As with any business, continued over-drawing and uncontrolled debt will eventually be stopped by the bank which will refuse to honour cheques and standing orders.

Dr White gave the other partners in her South London practice 12 months notice that she intended to leave. She planned to withdraw the money she had left in the practice to fund a years' travelling. During her final year, the practice list size reduced significantly with a corresponding reduction in profits. The partners' drawings were not adjusted, and as a result when the year-end accounts were compiled, they showed that Dr White was significantly over-drawn. The funds she assumed would be paid out to her on her retirement had to be used to repay this over-drawing. This left her without the funds for her travels.

Further points worth clarifying about the balance sheet include the following:
- Fixed assets are so called because they are expected to have a life of more than one year. Typically these will include premises where the practice owns the building, fixtures, fittings and equipment such as computers. These assets will appear in each balance sheet, but they will also wear out and lose value. This process, known as 'depreciation', is demonstrated in the accounts by transferring part of the asset to an expense in the profit and loss account. In the accounts above, you can see on the balance sheet the fixed assets have fallen from £3,720 to £3,162 showing the fall in value of the

assets. The profit and loss account shows a corresponding expense of £558 which represents the fall in value as an expense.

- Figures shown in brackets such as (£1,000) are an accountant's way of recording a negative number. GPs do occasionally misunderstand this use of parentheses and mistake liabilities for assets.

The bottom section on the balance sheet is the capital accounts, also known as the current accounts. The capital accounts represent each partner's share of the net assets.

Assets – Liabilities = Capital, which means there is a direct link between what happens on one side of the equation and what happens on the other. If the capital has changed, so must the assets and/or the liabilities. This means that if a partner under-draws, in other words their drawings are less than their profit share, there will be more assets left in the practice, and that partner's capital/current account will increase. Therefore, in a partnership with a number of partners, each with their own capital account, as each partner either under- or over-draws, so the net assets go up and down and each partner's capital account will change to reflect this.

In the Sunnihill accounts, Dr Ghode has seen his capital account decrease from £27,580 to £25,304, a decrease of £2,276. Dr Stern has seen his account fall from £33,866 to £21,856, a fall of £12,010, and Dr Hart from £17,965 to £14,712, a fall of £3,253. In the absence of any kind of explanation, this would cause concern. Falling net assets suggest the partners are over-drawing. However, every case needs to be looked at critically: while the partners did over-draw in this year, they did have the resources available. At the beginning of the year, they had £79,411 in the practice which has fallen to £61,872. That amount in itself does not cause the practice a difficulty as it is still solvent, but it could become insolvent within a few years if the trend is not reversed.

5

SUNNIHILL HEALTH CENTRE
SCHEDULES OF INCOME
FOR THE YEAR ENDED 31 MARCH 2010

	Sch	2010 £	2009 £
SCHEDULE 1			
Fees Earned			
Global Sum		341,241	329,254
Staff		–	1,000
Less: Opt-out Out of Hours		(20,206)	(20,973)
Correction Factor		80,910	91,637
Seniority		9,581	8,394
		411,526	409,312
Quality and Outcome Framework	4	112,096	99,767
Enhanced Services	5	45,245	40,018
		568,867	549,097
Registered List		6,255	6,481
Weighted List		5,884	6,097
SCHEDULE 2			
Reimbursements			
Locums		21,187	(533)
Rent and Rates		24,480	24,000
Computer Expenses		–	4,848
Drugs		19,638	15,767
		65,305	44,082

6

SUNNIHILL HEALTH CENTRE
SCHEDULES OF INCOME
FOR THE YEAR ENDED 31 MARCH 2010

	2010 £	2009 £
SCHEDULE 3		
Other Income		
Superannuable		
Student Doctor Training	2,198	–
Non-Superannuable		
Private Fees	12,790	11,236
Bank Deposit Interest	1,618	865
	16,606	12,101

SCHEDULE 4

Quality and Outcome Framework

	2010		Maximum	2009	
	Total £	Number of points	Points Available	Total £	Number of points
Clinical Domain	68,463	653	655	62,514	646
Organisational	21,122	160	181	16,797	140
Additional Services	5,584	36	36	5,025	36
Patient Experience	14,283	108	108	12,919	108
Holistic Care	2,644	20	20	2,512	19
	112,096	977	1,000	99,767	949

7

SUNNIHILL HEALTH CENTRE
SCHEDULES OF INCOME
FOR THE YEAR ENDED 31 MARCH 2010

	2010 £	2009 £
SCHEDULE 5		
Enhanced Services		
Directed Enhanced Services		
Improved Access Scheme	11,083	6,127
Childhood Immunisation Targets	5,241	10,495
Influenza	5,337	6,089
Minor Surgery	362	1,556
Phlebotomy	1,298	748
Information Management and Technology	(37)	2,635
Choose and Book	5,387	–
Post-Operative Care	1,380	2,741
National Enhanced Services		
IUCD Fitting	2,073	2,648
Drug Misuse	813	800
Smoking Cessation	–	965
Local Enhanced Services		
Practice Based Commissioning	11,385	5,214
Methotrexate	563	–
SMEP	360	–
	45,245	40,018

8

SUNNIHILL HEALTH CENTRE
NOTES TO THE ACCOUNTS
FOR THE YEAR ENDED 31 MARCH 2010

1. ALLOCATION OF PROFIT

	Dr. G. £	Dr. S. £	Dr. H. £	Total £
Prior Allocation				
Seniority	6,926	1,969	686	9,581
Balance				
33.30: 44.40: 22.30	73,895	98,526	49,485	221,906
	80,821	100,495	50,171	231,487

Pages 5–7: Breakdown of income

These pages provide more background information to facilitate a better understanding of the accounts. Some accountants will include many pages, and some fewer. To be helpful they should be tailored to the needs of the individual practice.

Page 8: Allocation of profit

This page demonstrates how practice profits are divided between the partners and the workings behind these shares. Some income such as rental may be specific to only those partners who own the surgery. Similarly, some practice expenses such as locum insurance may differ between partners. This page is very important for two key reasons: firstly it determines how much each partner will earn, and secondly it will determine how much tax each partner will pay because UK tax is paid on a partner's profit.

Drs Brown, Marshall and Godson agreed that each partner would be paid an element of seniority, depending on how long they had been in general practice. Initially they planned this amount should be the same as the NHS paid to the practice as a seniority allowance, which was in the region of £7,000. However, the senior partner, Dr Brown, subsequently felt this amount was inadequate and unilaterally decided that £44,000 was more in line with his perception of his seniority. It may be obvious, but this automatically depleted the remaining profits for the other partners. If Dr Brown had taken an additional £37,000, Drs Marshall and Godson would each have been deprived of £18,500 worth of profits. In a frank discussion this was pointed out to Dr Brown who dropped his claim.

9

SUNNIHILL HEALTH CENTRE
NOTES TO THE ACCOUNTS
FOR THE YEAR ENDED 31 MARCH 2010

3. CURRENT ACCOUNTS

	Dr. G. £	Dr. S. £	Dr. H. £	Total £
Balance at 1 April 2009	27,580	33,866	17,965	79,411
Share of Profit	80,821	100,495	50,171	231,487
	108,401	134,361	68,136	310,898
Less:				
Drawings	45,500	53,800	31,560	130,860
Superannuation	13,775	21,475	8,033	43,283
Taxation	23,822	37,230	13,831	74,883
	83,097	112,505	53,424	249,026
Balance at 31 March 2010	25,304	21,856	14,712	61,872

10

SUNNIHILL HEALTH CENTRE
SCHEDULE OF DRAWINGS
FOR THE YEAR ENDED 31 MARCH 2010

	Dr. G. £	Dr. S. £	Dr. H. £	Total £
MONTH				
April	3,250	3,900	2,300	9,450
May	3,250	3,900	2,300	9,450
June	3,600	4,100	2,500	10,200
July	3,600	4,100	2,500	10,200
August	3,600	4,100	2,500	10,200
September	3,600	4,100	2,500	10,200
October	3,600	4,100	2,500	10,200
November	3,600	4,100	2,500	10,200
December	3,600	4,200	2,500	10,300
January	1,800	2,100	1,250	5,150
February	1,800	2,100	1,250	5,150
March	1,800	2,100	1,250	5,150
	37,100	42,900	25,850	105,850
Additional Drawings	8,400	10,900	5,710	25,010
	45,500	53,800	31,560	130,860

Pages 9 and 10: Current accounts and drawings

These pages show the movement on each partner's current or capital account. Each partner starts with the balance they left in last year which is increased by their profit share for the year. The amount of money or drawings they have taken out of the practice, their pension contributions or superannuation and any other personal expense they may have are then deducted. In the Sunnihill partnership the practice pays the partners' tax, so it is included in this section.

A note about partnership taxation
Until 1996–1997, partnership tax was separately calculated by HMRC and paid by the partnership. It was a joint and several liability, which meant that if one partner refused or was unable to pay their tax, HMRC could sue the other partners for the tax. For this reason, many practices collected the tax in the practice and paid HMRC directly, avoiding the possibility of a partner not paying their tax. Since 1996–1997 there is no joint and several liability, and in most cases partners take out their drawings 'gross' and pay their own tax. Some partners prefer to leave the responsibility for paying their tax to the partnership, and continue on the same basis as before. There is no right or wrong choice, but if a partner has other income or wealth, they will have a further tax liability, and a compensatory adjustment which reduces their drawings will need to be made. Paying the tax through the practice can significantly increase or decrease the capital accounts, making constant adjustment a necessary process. The rules for limited companies are different, but in principle through the use of partnerships the partners pay income tax on their share of the profits. The partnership does not exist in legal terms as a separate legal entity, and no partnership tax is charged. Limited companies do exist in their own right and pay corporation tax on the profits.

11

SUNNIHILL HEALTH CENTRE
FOR THE YEAR ENDED 31 MARCH 2010
PRACTICE STATISTICS

	Ramsay Brown Guide	2010	2009
Staff Wages Efficiency Ratio	33.00%	$\frac{189,588}{568,867} = 33.33\%$	$\frac{166,547}{549,097} = 30.33\%$
Clinical Assistance Ratio	14.00%	$\frac{128,232}{568,867} = 22.54\%$	$\frac{88,146}{549,097} = 16.05\%$
Administrative Ratio	7.56%	$\frac{28,464}{568,867} = 5.00\%$	$\frac{33,294}{549,097} = 6.06\%$
Financial and Professional Ratio	1.75%	$\frac{9,226}{568,867} = 1.62\%$	$\frac{6,249}{549,097} = 1.14\%$
New Contract Income per Patient Ratio	£110.00	$\frac{568,867}{6,255} = £90.95$	$\frac{549,097}{5,775} = £95.08$
Global Sum Equivalent plus Seniority	£79.00	$\frac{411,526}{6,255} = £65.79$	$\frac{408,312}{5,775} = £70.70$
Quality and Outcome Framework Income	£18.00	$\frac{112,096}{6,255} = £17.92$	$\frac{99,767}{5,775} = £17.28$
Enhanced Services Income	£12.50	$\frac{45,245}{6,255} = £7.23$	$\frac{40,018}{5,775} = £6.93$
Other Income per Patient Ratio	£9.00	$\frac{16,606}{6,255} = £2.65$	$\frac{12,101}{5,775} = £2.10$
Net Profit per Patient Ratio	£55.00	$\frac{231,487}{6,255} = £37.01$	$\frac{267,493}{5,775} = £46.32$
Net Profit per Partner	£133,500	$\frac{231,487}{2.25} = £102,833$	$\frac{267,493}{2.25} = £118,885$

12

SUNNIHILL HEALTH CENTRE
FOR THE YEAR ENDED 31 MARCH 2010
PRACTICE STATISTICS WORKINGS

	2010 £	2009 £
Staff Wages Efficiency Ratio		
Salaries and Wages	173,112	150,652
Note Summarising	6,506	5,270
Staff Welfare	3,157	3,701
Staff Pension	6,787	5,784
Staff Training	26	1,140
	189,588	166,547
Clinical Assistance Ratio		
Salaried Assistant (Net)	101,462	68,684
Locums (Net)	24,853	18,396
Deputising and Co-op Service	1,917	1,066
	128,232	88,146
Administrative Ratio		
Health Centre Charges	–	10,782
Telephone	6,557	5,119
Computer Expenses (Net)	1,580	1,425
Printing, Postage and Stationery	8,068	6,749
General Expenses	147	151
Hire of Equipment	516	473
Courses and Conferences	424	–
Advertising	869	361
Travelling	184	207
Repairs and Maintenance	2,589	700
Insurance	1,150	969
Parking Permit Change	2,315	2,920
Levies	3,507	2,782
Depreciation – Medical Equipment	316	371
Depreciation – Fixtures and Fittings	242	285
	28,464	33,294
Financial and Professional Ratio		
Bank Interest and Charges	914	239
Legal and Professional Fees	3,612	1,533
Accountancy	4,700	4,477
	9,226	6,249

Pages 11 and 12: Practice statistics

These key ratios show how much of the core NHS practice income, that is income which excludes any private fees or reimbursements, is spent running the practice and how much core income is generated per patient. No two practices are the same, but this exercise provides a guide and a range. A practice outside the range merits further examination.

There are several key ratios dealing with the expenses of the practice; these are discussed next, starting with the four most important ratios.

1. Staff efficiency ratio

This shows how much of the practice's core NHS income is spent on staff. This includes the following expenses:

1 Gross salary costs of the management, reception, secretarial and nursing.
2 Pension costs relating to the staff in (1).
3 Staff training and recruitment costs.

Typically these costs will range from 25% to 35% of core NHS income. These figures will vary from practice to practice depending on factors such as the use of nurses to cover GP sessions or whether the practice income is high or low as the denominator will affect the percentage. Nevertheless, this ratio is an important measure of the efficiency of the staff and is most valuable when used as a comparative measure against the percentages from previous years.

Where the percentage is high, and in rare cases it has been known to reach 90%, partners would benefit from understanding why. An outside consultant can help to determine how staff are working to affect this ratio.

In the Sunnihill accounts, 33.3% of core income is spent on staff, which is within an acceptable range.

2. Clinical assistance ratio

This ratio looks at the amount of the NHS core practice income which is used to fund extra nonpartner GP help such as locums and salaried GPs together with their deputising costs. If the practice is reimbursed for any of these costs, then only the net costs are taken into account. Typically these costs are around 14% of the core NHS income. This percentage works on the premise that the average GP principal has 2,500 patients, so if the practice had one principal and 5,000 patients, an acceptable percentage would be twice the average at 28%.

The Sunnihill practice spends 22.54% of its core NHS income on salaried assistants and locums. The list size is 6,255, and there are 2.25 full time principals (i.e. 2,780 patients per principal). An acceptable percentage cost would be around 15.58% (i.e. 14% × 2780/2500), making the cost of 22.54% unacceptable.

3. Administrative expenses ratio
This ratio looks at how much core NHS income is spent on the day to day running costs for the practice. Once again, any reimbursements are deducted from these costs. A typical list of these expenses includes the following:
Health centre charges
Telephones
Computer expenses (net)
Printing, postage and stationery
General expenses
Hire of equipment
Courses and conferences
Advertising
Travelling
Repairs and maintenance
Insurance
Parking permit change
Levies
Depreciation – medical equipment
Depreciation – fixtures and fittings
Typically, these costs are around 7.5% of core NHS income, but they will vary depending on the practice location and whether it has branch surgeries. Again, the measure is most useful when compared with previous years.

These ratios provide an effective tool for assessing the accuracy of projected costs.

Partners at the Orange practice were offered the chance to move to a new purpose built NHS premises. They would no longer have to pay health centre charges of £6,000 but would have to pay a service charge of £40,000 per annum in addition to all their existing costs. This increased their costs from 5% to more than 12%. Armed with this information, the partners were able to negotiate with the primary care trust (PCT) and limit the costs to 6% of core NHS income.

The Sunnihill practice spends an acceptable 5% of its core income on administrative expenses.

4. Financial and professional ratio
This ratio examines the proportion of core NHS income spent on accountancy, legal, other professional and banking fees, excluding mortgage interest. The average percentage is around 1.75%. The Sunnyhill practice spends 1.62%.

5. New contract income per patient
This shows the amount of earnings per patient either from the 2004 General Medical Services (GMS) contract or from the practice's Personal Medical

Services (PMS) or Alternative Providers of Medical Services (APMS) contract. It comprises the total of the next income ratios.

6. Global sum equivalent/baseline, plus seniority

This ratio looks at the core income the practice receives mainly from the number of patients on the list. It varies considerably between practices, but once set it remains fairly constant unless there is an attempt to restructure the basis of payment. The amount per patient ranges from £65 to £140. This ratio is key when considering the effect of changes on partners' profits: a practice earning £65 per patient is limited in how much it can change without impacting directly on partners' profits. In contrast, a practice which is earning £130 per patient and facing a reduction to £110 can make changes with a minimal reduction of the partners' profits.

The Sunnihill practice earns £65 per patient, which is close to the lowest range. This means that there is very little room for manoeuvre. Having limited resources means that the partners have limited options as to how they run the practice. A healthy supply of income allows the partners more flexibility in the way they manage the practice.

7. Quality and outcome framework income

This ratio shows how much the practice earns from the 2004 New Contract Quality and Outcomes Framework. The average is around £18.00, and Sunnihill achieved £17.92.

8. Enhanced services income ratio

This ratio shows how much the practice earns from the 2004 New Contract Enhanced Services. The average is around £12.50, and Sunnihill achieved £7.23. There are three possible explanations for this: firstly the practice may have chosen not to do the enhanced services, secondly the PCT may not be offering the enhanced services as there is a considerable variation between PCTs or thirdly the practice may be doing the work but not claiming properly.

9. Net profit per patient ratio

This key ratio shows the net profit per patient. The average is close to £55 per patient. Sunnihill only achieved £37.01, which merits an explanation: should a partner leave and be replaced with a salaried assistant, the cost of the salaried assistant will appear as an expense in the profit and loss account, reducing the overall profits and the £ per patient. In the Sunnihill practice, a partner left with a resultant decrease in the number of principals. This meant reduced profits were shared between fewer partners, so the reduction in profits per patient would be expected although the profit per partner may increase.

This ratio is important when the figure is unexpected and is also an indicator of a trend.

10. Net profit per partner ratio
This key figure is the net profit that each partner earns from the practice.

Partners can request useful information from the accounts

The ratios listed above are all important, some more than others. The first four expense ratios will always be relevant, regardless of the contract GPs are working to. The new contract income ratios are likely to change depending on the funding streams available. They are included here to highlight what information can be extrapolated from the accounts and which GPs can rightly ask their managers and accountants to provide to them. The last two ratios, net profit per patient and per partner, are not time dependent and will always provide GPs with important and critical information.

Having this kind of information arms GPs with the financial intelligence necessary to quantitatively assess the practice. A full set of accounts as they appear in practice is included in Appendix 2.

When Dr Grey was invited to join the Central practice, he requested a set of accounts and was given the following financial information:

The Central Practice
Year Ended 30 September 2009

Core NHS Income		£2,245,038
Other Income		196,142
Total Income		2,441,180
Less		
Drugs and Instruments	£18,160	
Locum Costs	793,156	
Deputising Costs	11,936	
Training Costs	8,476	
Staff Salaries	1,209,912	
Heat and Light	44,534	
Insurance	11,878	
Cleaning	44,020	
Repairs	7,118	
Computer Expenses	12,532	
Telephone	46,416	
Subscriptions	34,734	
Advertising	6,234	
Printing, Postage and Stationery	29,362	
Accountancy	22,326	
Legal and Professional Fees	17,400	
Bank Charges and Interest	4,100	
LMC Levies	12,354	
General Expenses	10,726	£2,345,374
Net Profit		£95,806

The Central practice had four full time partners and a list size of 26,000 patients. Each partner earned £23,950. In addition, each partner's capital account was over-drawn by almost £90,000, and the practice was in significant debt. At first glance Dr Grey or indeed any prospective partner should walk away from this low profit, insolvent practice. However, the ratio analysis revealed a different picture:

The Central Practice
For the Year Ended 30 September 2009
Practice Statistics

	Guide	Actual
Staff Wages Efficiency Ratio	33.00%	$\dfrac{1,218,388}{2,245,038} = 54.27\%$
Clinical Assistance Ratio	14.00%	$\dfrac{805,092}{2,245,038} = 35.86\%$
Administrative Ratio	7.50%	$\dfrac{278,068}{2,245,038} = 12.38\%$
Financial and Professional Ratio	1.75%	$\dfrac{43,826}{2,245,038} = 1.95\%$
New Contract Income per Patient Ratio	£110.00	$\dfrac{2,245,038}{26,000} = £86.34$
Other Income per Patient Ratio	£9.00	$\dfrac{196,142}{6,255} = £31.35$
Net Profit per Patient Ratio	£55.00	$\dfrac{95,806}{26,000} = £3.84$
Net Profit per Partner	£33,500	$\dfrac{95,806}{4.00} = £23,951$

The ratios highlighted two key problems: firstly that the practice had less income than average and secondly that it spent an excessive amount on locums and staff.

On first appraisal, this practice should have spent 33% of its core income on staff costs; indeed, as a larger practice, economies of scale make 33% quite generous. At 54.37%, the practice annually over-spent £477,525.

The average practice spends 14% of its income on clinical assistance (i.e. salaried GPs, locums and deputising services). The average practice has approximately 2,500 patients per principal. The Central practice has 26,000 patients and 4 partners (i.e. 6,500 patients per principal). Therefore the target percentage for clinical assistance needs to be amended to 36.4% (14% × 6500/2500). Adjusting the target in this way makes the spend of 35.86% appear reasonable.

The average administrative ratio is 7.5%. At 12.3% this amounts to a £109,690 overspend. Again, economies of scale should enable this larger practice to function at a lower than average ratio.

The financial and professional ratio is close enough to average to leave alone.

The lower than average income per patient is a major cause for concern. A practice can change its expenses, but it is far harder to change the income per patient which is contractually set by the NHS. At £86.34, the Central practice is forced to manage on less revenue than the average practice.

The following financial scenario shows what would happen if the Central practice ratios were adjusted to the national average:

Profits for the year ended 30 September 2009	£95,806.00
Add	
Overspending on staff	£477,525.00
Overspending on administrative expenses	£109,690.00
	£683,021.00
Profits per partner	£170,755.00

This is a dramatic but achievable improvement, not least because it brings the practice in line with others. However, as with many business changes, achieving these numbers involves making and executing difficult decisions.

Using the above comparisons, Dr Grey explained to the other partners that the practice was falling short on its potential. She agreed to join them on the condition that she was allowed to drive through the necessary changes to raise the profits. This involved large scale redundancies, the reallocation of responsibilities and a critical review of the services brought in by the practice The staff changes were painful initially, but at the same time the practice became more efficient, so the patients and partners did not notice any failings. By the end of the first year the partners' over-drawings had reduced dramatically and the whole practice had become stronger.

Capital and current accounts

This part of the accounts is more likely to cause confusion than any other. It is important because it sets out how much each partner in the practice owns of the net assets. This is key for two reasons:

1 It sets out how much each partner is entitled to at the date of the balance sheet, and that entitlement crystallises when a partner leaves the practice by either death or retirement.

2 It sets out how much of the net assets that partner has left in the practice relative to the other partners.

As already stated, the terms 'capital account' and 'current account' are synonymous. In the Sunnihill accounts the net assets are set out in the balance sheet followed by the partners' current accounts which might also be called the capital account. How they are labelled is not important, but what they represent is. Some accountants like to use more than one set of capital or current accounts, particularly if some of the assets are owned in different shares. This is the case in the following example:

West Surgery
Balance Sheet as at 31 March 2010

	Note	2010 £		2009 £	
Fixed Assets					
Property		383,487		383,487	
Less Mortgage		(256,659)		(278,032)	
		126,828		105,455	
Tangible Assets		10,074		11,851	
		136,902		117,306	
Current Assets					
Stock of Drugs		1,813		1,961	
Sundry Debtors and Prepayments		76,622		94,075	
GP Monies		2,091		2,090	
Main Bank Account		43,210		11,268	
Petty Cash		821		156	
		124,557		109,550	
Current Liabilities					
Superannuation		13,401		8,384	
Sundry Creditors and Accruals		22,084		32,949	
		35,485		41,333	
Net Current Assets			89,072		68,217
			225,974		185,523
Represented By					
Property Capital Accounts			126,828		105,455
Other Asset Capital Accounts			55,000		55,000
Current Accounts			44,146		25,068
			225,974		185,523

The Problems with differential current accounts

Drs Smith and Levy share profits equally, but their capital accounts are as shown:

	Dr Smith £	Dr Jones £	Total £
Balance brought forward	5,000	25,000	30,000
Profit for the year	120,000	120,000	240,000
	125,000	145,000	270,000
Less drawings	− 115,000	− 90,000	− 205,000
	10,000	55,000	65,000

The practice has net assets of £65,000 meaning there is little cause for concern at a top-line level. Should Dr Smith leave he would be entitled to £10,000, while if Dr Levy were to leave he would expect £55,000. However, at a personal level it is probably unfair that Dr Levy has £55,000 of his wealth tied up in the practice, while Dr Smith has only £10,000. Dr Levy cannot access his money because Dr Smith has a relatively small amount deposited in the practice. This could be resolved if Dr Smith injected £22,500 and Dr Levy withdrew £22,500, but it would be unwise for Dr Smith to simply give Dr Levy the money outside the accounts. This is because if the transaction does not appear in the accounts, the £22,500 discrepancy will still exist in the following years. For clarity, the introduction and withdrawal of funds must be paid in, and then out, of the practice accounts.

Some GPs believe that any money remaining in the capital accounts at the financial year-end should be withdrawn, leaving a zero balance. This means the net assets would be zero, which is unwise. Running a practice without any reserve leaves it financially vulnerable to the smallest hiccup, be that a delay in receiving income or an unplanned expense.

No apples ever kept the taxman at bay

Any business person understands the need to keep up to date with their taxation obligations. For a self-employed doctor, it is vital. This is not just for their personal peace of mind or even the security of the practice, but also because their professional standing depends on being blemish free. If the HMRC finds against a doctor, they will be reported to the General Medical Council (GMC).

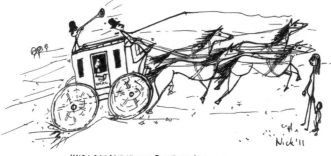

HMRC ARE NOT KNOWN FOR THEIR PATIENCE

HMRC are not known for their patience in waiting for payments, which makes it important to set aside sufficient monies to pay the tax when it is due. Those who have been GPs for years will know when their tax is due, but a newly appointed GP will commonly pay no tax for 18 months and then find themselves facing a single payment for the whole period:

Dr Crow joined the Ivory practice as a partner on 1 April 2007. She was advised that her first tax liability would not arise for several months and she should put aside 35% of her income. By October 2008, Dr Crow had not received any tax demands and used the money she had put aside to buy a new car. On 15 January 2009 she received a demand from HMRC for £31,200 but only had £5,000 left in the account. Dr Crow had no means of raising the additional funds by the due date, 31 January 2009, and the practice had to lend her the money to pay the tax.

The practice accountant can advise on how much tax to put aside to meet tax liabilities. As a rule of thumb, putting 35% of any income received into a separate account should provide sufficient funds to meet most tax bills.

Key points

- Your practice accounting system must be tailored to meet your needs.
- If your staff do not understand double entry bookkeeping, select a simpler system.
- Understanding your accounts helps you to stay on top of your practice.
- Fixed assets are expected to last more than one year.
- Current assets are expected to turn into liquid funds within 12 months.
- Current liabilities are those debts expected to be paid within 12 months.
- Capital and current accounts are synonymous and refer to the amount of wealth owned by each partner.

- If the net asset value of a practice increases, so will the partner's capital or current accounts.
- Ratio analysis can be used to set and control practice expenditure.
- Capital or current accounts should be in proportion to ownership of assets and profit sharing ratio.

Chapter 4 **Budgeting**

Accounting is the process of reporting past financial information in a meaningful way. It is by definition historic and summarizes what has happened rather than what will or may happen.

Budgeting is an exercise in looking forward and planning, based on experience and past history. It is impossible to predict the final figures with certainty, but the process of budgeting focuses GP partners on the trends affecting the practice, and therefore the plans they need to make for the future. Working to a budget also enables GPs to identify the impact of sudden changes in revenues or costs and therefore make changes to mitigate against these:

Partners drawings at the Violet practice were £5,000 per partner per month. In the year to 31 March 2010, the PCT conducted a list cleaning exercise and wrote to the whole list. Any non-responsive patients were immediately removed, and the practice lost 1,500 of its 9,000 total. The financial impact was catastrophic as monthly global sum payments of £8,125, quarterly enhanced services of £3,750 and a final reduced Quality and Outcome Framework (QOF) payment of £28,165 were cut. Neither the partners nor the practice manager could bear to look at the outcomes, and the practice blindly continued drawing their £5,000 per month.

After five months, the cash reserves ran out and the bank refused to honour cheques. The partners were forced to reduce their drawings and take a bank loan at a prohibitive rate.

Had the partners been used to budgeting, they could have predicted the impact of the reduced income, looked at what they could do to mitigate against this and also negotiated a loan with the bank from a position of

How to Manage Your GP Practice, First Edition. Farine Clarke and Laurence Slavin.
© 2012 John Wiley & Sons, Ltd. Published 2012 by John Wiley & Sons, Ltd.

strength. Indeed a well organised small business would have started this process the minute they knew the PCT exercise was underway, and mapped out a 'best case' and 'worst case' scenario to prepare for difficulties ahead. Banks prefer to loan to people they consider are on top of their finances, even if those clients have hit a misfortune.

Budgeting can be as simple as a basic calculation for the next year's events, or a monthly or even daily estimate of likely incomes and expenses.

The following is a simple example:

Dr Kirker compiled his budget with his accountant. He had 2,000 patients, a global sum of £65 per patient, 900 QOF points, enhanced services at £10 per patient and teaching income and private fees of £10,000.

Based on his previous year, he estimated his staff costs at £50,000, locum costs at £25,000 and running costs of £25,000.

This produced the following top-line budget:

Global sum	£130,000
QOF	38,195
Enhanced services	20,000
Other income	10,000
	198,195
Less	
Staff costs	50,000
Locum costs	25,000
Running costs	25,000
Profit	98,195

Knowing the practice made £98,195 was useful overall but limiting as a day to day management tool. Dr Kirker assumed that he could safely draw £8,000 a month against his profit figure until his accountant pointed out that 30% of the QOF was paid at the end of the financial year and the enhanced services payment was quarterly. To clarify the position, he presented the data on a monthly basis to Dr Kirker, whose accounting year ran from April 1 to March 31 (Table 4.1).

The spreadsheet showed that if Dr Kirker drew £8,000 per month, the practice would be overdrawn for eight months and close to zero for three. The practice did not have sufficient money in reserve to accommodate these peaks and troughs, and the funds were only replenished by a cash injection in March of the final QOF payment. Clearly Dr Kirker had to manage his drawings in line with the overall cash flow of the practice.

Table 4.1 Dr Kirker monthly budget

	April	May	June	July	Aug	Sept	Oct	Nov	Dec	Jan	Feb	Mar
Global sum	£10,833	£10,833	£10,834	£10,833	£10,833	£10,834	£10,833	£10,833	£10,834	£10,833	£10,833	£10,834
QOF	2,228	2,228	2,228	2,228	2,228	2,228	2,228	2,228	2,228	2,228	2,228	13,687
Enhanced services	0	0	5,000	0	0	5,000	0	0	5,000	0	0	5,000
Other income	833	833	834	833	833	834	833	833	834	833	833	834
Total income	13,894	13,894	18,896	13,894	13,894	18,896	13,894	13,894	18,896	13,894	13,894	30,355
Salaries	4,167	4,167	4,166	4,167	4,167	4,166	4,167	4,167	4,166	4,167	4,167	4,166
Locum costs	2,083	2,083	2,084	2,083	2,083	2,084	2,083	2,083	2,084	2,083	2,083	2,084
Running costs	2,083	2,083	2,084	2,083	2,083	2,084	2,083	2,083	2,084	2,083	2,083	2,084
Total costs	8,333	8,333	8,334	8,333	8,333	8,334	8,333	8,333	8,334	8,333	8,333	8,334
Monthly surplus	5,561	5,561	10,562	5,561	5,561	10,562	5,561	5,561	10,562	5,561	5,561	22,021

The initial projected profit of £98,195 is a top-line budget for the year, and the monthly calculations are a cash flow forecast mirroring what is expected to happen to the bank balance. Therefore the budgeting process involves firstly determining the top-line profit and loss, and then predicting the timing of revenue and costs on a monthly basis, the so-called phased budget. The actual figures are not always exactly as predicted and therefore need to be monitored against the real figures each month. This is good practice because it helps the partners understand on a monthly basis exactly what is happening to their cash flow, which in turn enables them to adapt the practice activities accordingly.

For example, if the practice sent its enhanced services claims in late, its list size increased by 200 patients between setting the budget and the start of the new financial year and staff costs included a £3,000 unbudgeted bonus in June, the effect would be as in Table 4.2.

As long as Dr Kirker monitored his accounts against his budget, he could take steps such as delaying the bonus payment or even chasing his enhanced service payments to reduce the negative impact against budget in June.

Good businesses compile good budgets

In commercial businesses the finance director usually takes the lead to compile company budgets each year. He or she will ask all the directors to contribute to the process, and they in turn will gain information from their front-line staff and third parties, such as suppliers. Depending on the size and area of the business, budgeting can begin several months or even a year before it becomes live and it will follow a strict budget timetable. Good budgeting is essential for a successful business, which means the process is taken very seriously. Evolving budgets are subject to intense scrutiny and will often be revised several times before being granted final approval by the board.

To compile a budget, company directors will first make a series of assumptions about every element which constitutes the revenue and costs. By definition these assumptions will not be 100% accurate, but they are based on business expertise, what happened the previous year and changes in the marketplace. Fixed costs are relatively straightforward to predict, but variables, particularly in revenue, are more difficult. For example, businesses which sell products will depend on the 'market' for their revenue, which in turn may be determined by demographic changes and the economy overall. The keener the directors' understanding of the market in which they function, the more accurate their budget will be.

Many businesses will also prepare 'what if' scenario budgets at this stage, to show what will happen to the profit if one or more key factors change in their

Table 4.2 Dr Kirker updated monthly budget

	April budget	April actual	April variance	May budget	May actual	May variance	June budget	June actual	June variance
Global sum	£10,833	£11,916	£1,083	10,833	£11,916	£1,083	10,833	£11,916	£1,083
QOF	2,228	2,228	0	2,228	2,228	0	2,228	2,228	0
Enhanced services	0	0	0	0	0	0	5,000	0	–5,000
Other income	833	833	0	833	833	0	833	833	0
Total income	13,894	14,977	1,083	13,894	14,977	1,083	18,894	14,977	–3,917
Salaries	4,167	4,167	0	4,167	4,167	0	4,167	7,167	3,000
Locum costs	2,083	2,083	0	2,083	2,083	0	2,083	2,083	0
Running costs	2,083	2,083	0	2,083	2,083	0	2,083	2,083	0
Total costs	8,333	8,333	0	8,333	8,333	0	8,333	11,333	3,000
Monthly variance		1083			1083			3,000	–6917

assumptions. For example, what will happen to the profit if the market shrinks by 20%, or if the price of a vital manufacturing material increases by 15%? Or, how will cutting the salary bill by 10% impact the business in terms of revenue, costs and profit? This not only gives directors a sense of the danger areas and the opportunity to consider new plans for the business, but also helps to mitigate against one of the key downfalls of many businesses, namely over-optimistic budgeting. This can take many forms, but the most common is where directors or their staff over-estimate the revenues and underestimate the costs. This combined effect makes the projected profits far greater than they are in reality. Directors will also take soundings from their departmental staff when making assumptions for the budget. They usually know which members of staff are financial optimists and which are pessimists, and will temper the figures they put into the budget accordingly.

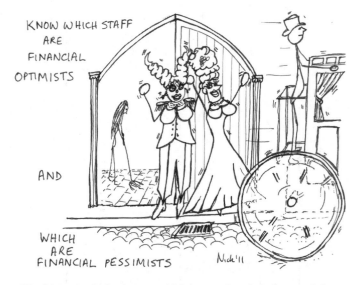

KNOW WHICH STAFF ARE FINANCIAL OPTIMISTS

AND

WHICH ARE FINANCIAL PESSIMISTS

Nick'11

Difficulties arise for businesses which have enjoyed profit growth for many years, but are predicting changes which result in a budgeted profit that is lower than the previous year's. Commercial boards prefer to see year on year profit growth, and directors have a difficult job when presenting a budget which shows a fall. However they also know that simply making the budget look better in order to get it approved by the board is a short term strategy, as most boards view missing a budget once it is live as unforgivable failure.

Small business owners feel it is better to set a pessimistic budget and beat it, that is, exceed the budgeted profit rather than be over-optimistic and fail. Banks and other financial institutions prefer this when asked to lend money as they can have faith that the business is able to service its debts. Finance directors in commercial organisations have shareholders to satisfy and therefore tread a fine line between setting realistic budgets while maintaining shareholder value and confidence in the business.

In general practice, the most appropriate time to set the budget is as soon as the practice accounts have been prepared for the previous year. The practice accountant who is familiar with the finances and will have experience in compiling budgets can assist in the process.

Key points

- Good businesses compile useful budgets.
- Use the budgeting process to focus everyone's minds on the practice finances and plans.
- Accounts look at historic data; budgets build on that data to make informed predictions.
- Comparing monthly actuals with the monthly budget affords the opportunity to make timely changes.
- Cash flow forecasts predict the movement of liquid funds in the practice.
- Variance analysis tracks the variations between budgets and the actual results.
- Distinguishing between fixed and variable costs can help one make financial decisions.
- Budgeting for 'what if' scenarios can help to mitigate against unexpected events.

Chapter 5 **Choosing the right operational model for the practice**

The basic differences in business models were described in Chapter 3. The following flow chart helps to determine which model to adopt:

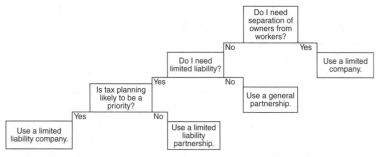

Figure 5.1 Operational model flowchart.

GP liability for debts or obligations

A limited company limits the amount for which a shareholder can be sued. This is usually the face value of the shares, and is often a nominal £1 per share. In a limited liability partnership, each partner's personal liability is limited to the amount that they have pledged to the partnership. Again this can be as little as £1. In a general partnership each partner is liable for partnership debts without limit and is jointly and severally liable with the other partners. This exposure can be covered by employers' liability insurance and professional indemnity insurance provided by organisations such as the Medical Defence Union (MDU), Medical Protection Society (MPS) and Medical and Dental Defence Union of Scotland (MDDUS). If a shareholder in a limited company

How to Manage Your GP Practice, First Edition. Farine Clarke and Laurence Slavin.
© 2012 John Wiley & Sons, Ltd. Published 2012 by John Wiley & Sons, Ltd.

or a member of a limited liability partnership has given personal guarantees to, for example, a lender or as part of a lease arrangement, this liability is not protected by the limited company or the limited liability partnership.

Additional stakeholders

Of the three models, only the limited liability company allows the separation of the owners or shareholders from those running the practice with day to day decisions namely, the directors. In return for holding a share of the ownership, the shareholders receive dividends voted by the directors. The directors are paid a salary for running the practice. Using different classes of shares, each with their own set of rights, provides flexibility when expanding the stakeholders in the practice:

The Maroon practice was set up by three partners who wanted to be able to recruit two salaried GPs with a greater interest in the organisation than they would typically be given. At the same time, the partners did not want to give away any ownership of the practice. They formed a limited company called the Maroon Practice Limited and appointed themselves as directors. They also became shareholders in the 'A' shares which assigned to them the ownership of the company, as well as its voting and income rights. Maroon Practice Limited then issued B shares to the salaried GPs which had rights to income but not to voting or ownership. This gave the original three GPs the ability to vote income by way of dividends to the salaried GPs without giving away any ownership of the company.

Making finances public

Both limited companies and limited liability partnerships are required to publish their accounts at Companies House, where they can be accessed by any member of the public for a nominal fee.

Forming a partnership, limited company or limited liability partnership

The legal definition of a partnership is 'two or more individuals carrying on a business in common with a view to profits'. Forming a partnership is straightforward once you have found suitable colleagues. A partnership agreement is advisable but not essential, and without one the 1890 Partnership Act will govern the partnership and the conduct of the individuals within it. Such a partnership is called 'a partnership at will'. The following example illustrates how GPs may unwittingly be working in a partnership:

Two GP practices in Barnsley, each comprising five partners, started working together to provide enhanced services to their patients. They regarded this as an informal arrangement, although they purchased equipment in a name covering all the GPs, and represented themselves as one organisation to the local community. Each of the two practices brought the profits from their share of the joint organisation into their own practices and declared these to HMRC as part of the individual practice profits. The HMRC looked at the income and deemed the combined organisation to be a partnership. Since the individual practices had declared their share of income to HMRC, there was no loss of revenue to the tax office. However, HMRC still fined the practices for failing to submit partnership tax returns. This amounted to £100 per partner, per return, per annum.

Setting up a partnership is relatively straightforward. All the practice requires is a bank account, and each partner signs the bank mandate and must be approved for money laundering purposes.

A limited company and a limited liability partnership are both distinct from the partners, and accordingly have to be created. This can be achieved by engaging an accountant or lawyer to form a new limited company or limited liability partnership with a name of choice, or by purchasing a ready made 'off the shelf' limited company or limited liability partnership from a formation agent. The agent will change the name of the organisation, replace the directors and shareholders and change the registered office to the chosen address. Buying from an agent is akin to buying a display model car with no mileage; it is not bespoke, but it is cheaper and quicker. The certificate of incorporation as well as the individual directors' details are required to open a bank account in the name of the limited company or limited liability partnership.

The vast majority of GPs practice as partnerships, but there is a growing trend towards limited companies, hence their inclusion in this book. The following key points are common to all limited company accounts:

- The format of the accounts is fixed. The headings and the descriptions are set in law in the Companies Act and cannot be changed. This means the headings in the accounts for a limited company GP practice will be exactly the same as for a manufacturing or a financial service company. In order to get around the rigidity of this approach, many accountants will add a bespoke section at the end off the accounts which makes them more useful for the GPs. Because limited company accounts are published and available for public view, these extra, commercially sensitive pages are often removed prior to publication.

- In a set of partnership accounts, the partners' remuneration is their profit share while their drawings is the money they take out of the practice to live on. On the balance sheet, the drawings are not accounted for as a practice expense but as an advance on their profit share. In a limited company, the GPs who own and manage the practice are potentially remunerated in two separate ways; a directors' salary for their work managing the company and a dividend as an additional share of profits. Some companies prefer to offer salaries instead of dividends and vice versa. It is important to understand the difference between the two: the directors' salary, unlike the partners' drawing, is shown as a company expense. The dividends are shown as a deduction from the reserves of the company. Therefore, the directors' salary has to be separated out when analysing the results of a company in order to fully understand the overall performance of a business.

GPs in partnerships have capital or current accounts which are the 'undrawn' funds left in the practice and eventually paid out to the partner when they leave. Because partnerships are not legal entities, any wealth left in a partnership belongs to the partners. This contrasts with limited companies, which are separate legal entities, meaning the capital belongs to the company. At its simplest level, a set of limited company accounts will have two elements replacing the partnership's capital and current accounts. The company will have a share capital section, and a profit and loss account. The share capital reflects the amount of money that the company received for the face value of the shares. For instance, if the company issued 1,000 shares with a nominal value of 50p, the share capital in the accounts will show £500. If the company had sold the 1,000 shares with a nominal value of 50p for £1.25, the share capital in the accounts will still show £500, and the 'premium' of 75p per share is shown in the share premium account. In this case, the value shown would be £750 in the share premium account. The profit and loss account is the accumulated profits (or losses) that remain in the company. Unless the directors choose to pay out these profits as salary to themselves or dividends to the shareholders, they remain the property of the company.

Partnerships do not pay tax, but the partners pay income tax on their share of the profits. By contrast, companies do pay corporation tax on their profits; this is after the directors' salary but before dividends. Corporation tax for small companies is currently 20%, which means that the dividends are paid out of profits that have already incurred 20% tax. The individual shareholder pays a further 20% tax if they are higher rate taxpayers. The lower rate of corporation tax and the use of dividends are often used to justify the use of companies in preference to partnerships, but this often reflects a misunderstanding of the issues involved.

In the following example, the two directors receive salaries of £15,000 each. These costs are not visible as they are included in expenses. The profit and loss account shows a profit after corporation tax of £33,524. If we take this figure, and add back the directors' salaries to the profits available after corporation tax, the two shareholders and directors between them have generated £48,524. It is this figure that is directly comparable to a GP's share of profits from a partnership. Since an average GP earns around £135,000 (at 2009–2010), it is evident when we look at this figure that for two full time working GPs these are disappointing results. In order to understand why the practice is underperforming, the GPs will need the same level of analytical analysis that formed part of the partnership accounts analyses earlier.

The company is insolvent. For both 2009 and 2010, the company had net liabilities. The company moved from its own premises in 2009 to rented accommodation in 2010, hence the reduction in fixed assets and loans. Nevertheless, it is still insolvent.

The directors need to be careful because although limited companies have limited liability status, if the directors continue to trade while they know the company is insolvent they can become personally liable for the company's debts.

BIG BIRD LIMITED
PROFIT AND LOSS ACCOUNT
YEAR ENDED
31 MARCH 2010

	Year ended 31 March 2010 £	Year ended 31 March 2009 £
Turnover	528,890	655,617
Less costs of sales	− 436,975	− 610,791
Gross profit	91,915	44,826
Administrative expenses	− 50,091	− 77,482
Operating profit and loss	41,824	− 32,656
Interest payable and other charges	0	− 19,204
Profit or loss on ordinary activities before taxation	41,824	− 51,860
Taxation on profit or loss on ordinary activities	− 8,300	0
Profit or loss for the year	33,524	− 51,860
Accumulated profits and losses brought forward	− 51,860	0
Accumulated profits and losses carried forward	− 18,336	− 51,860

BIG BIRD LIMITED
BALANCE SHEET
AS AT 31 MARCH 2010

		As at 31 March 2010 £		As at 31 March 2009 £
Fixed assets				
Tangible assets		10,133		344,158
Current assets				
Stock	3,165		0	
Debtors	44,141		45,282	
Cash at bank and in hand	771		150	
	48,077		45,432	
Creditor: amounts falling	− 64,084		− 214,434	
due within one year				
		− 16,007		− 169,002
		− 5,874		175,156
Creditor: amounts falling		− 12,460		− 227,014
after more than				
one year				
Deficiency of assets		− 18,334		− 51,858
Capital and reserves				
Called up share capital		2		2
Profit and loss account		− 18,336		− 51,860
Shareholders funds		− 18,334		− 51,858

Key points

- Consider the appropriateness of using different business models, general partnerships, limited liability partnerships or limited companies.
- Without a partnership agreement, the 1890 Partnership Act will govern the practice arrangement.
- A partner joining a practice will always have to contribute capital; the contribution made by each GP should be proportional to their profit share.

Chapter 6 **Business growth**

No business in whatever trade or profession stands still.

A successful business is under constant pressure to expand because of customer demand, while an unsuccessful one will lean towards contraction. The same principle applies in general practice. As with any business, a practice under pressure to grow needs active management throughout the expansion process to achieve a successful outcome. The vast majority of businesses fail in

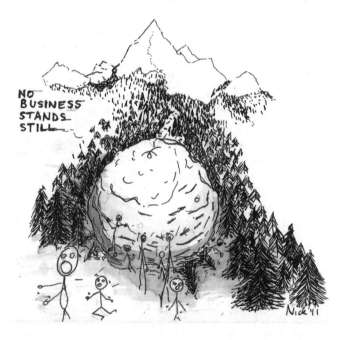

their early years because they are too 'successful', by which we mean they fall foul of a concept known as 'overtrading'. Simply put, the business launches with good products or services and is profitable, takes on more staff to meet growing demand and buys in more stocks thereby increasing the pressure on the cash flow. The expanding business sells more products or services but by the time the customers have paid their bills, the suppliers or core costs are overdue. This owed money can then put the company into liquidation. Many of these 'overtrading' businesses are consistently profitable, but they are simply unable to maintain their solvency.

Expansion should be linked to the vision partners have for their practice. If the practice is where the GPs want it to be, then expansion for the sake of it or because neighbouring practices are growing is probably unnecessary, unless of course the partners feel their own practice will be under increasing threat. Timing for expansion is also critical, and GPs should be comfortable that they have the time and resources to manage growth. Some businesses compile growth plans in advance to understand the scale of what is involved and then bring them forwards or tailor them as circumstances change.

Partners need to be sure that the effort involved in growth is worth it. They may need more GPs, more staff, new or extended premises and more equipment. They will certainly need more time and generate more work.

In 2009–2010, the average GP earned profits of £133,500. The highest earning GPs tended to be single-handed or two-partner practices with large list sizes (i.e. between 4,500 and 5,000 patients per partner). Typically this kind of practice employs locums, salaried GPs and nurses to help partners manage the large lists. If the partners' vision is to build the most profitable practice possible, then they are aiming for this model, namely one with the fewest number of partners and the largest list size. This is because the average GP principal earns approximately £14,000 per session after adjusting for superannuation and the average salaried GP costs £10,000 with on costs for superannuation and National Insurance. Opting for a salaried GP or locum instead of a partner generates profit.

If, on the other hand, the GPs want to build a practice based on long term relationships with their patients and the strongest possible reputation in the community, then they will aim for a model involving more partners caring for fewer patients. Of course the vast majority of GPs will want a combination of all the positive aspects of practice; good doctor–patient relationships, a strong reputation and reasonably high profits. There is no right or wrong, but knowing where the partners' emphasis lies will help them to devise the right growth plans for the practice.

Difficulties clearly arise when partners disagree about their end aims, which frequently happens, particularly when they are at different stages in their careers. In these circumstances it is prudent to try to reach an agreement as a partnership before any plans are drawn up. This also means that provision for those partners who do not wish to take part if, for example, they are near retirement can be made outside the plans without inhibiting their execution.

The following key issues are worth discussing in detail before embarking on a managed expansion plan:

• Methodology of expansion
• Clinical and patient need
• Staffing need
• Management
• Premises
• Funding
• Competition
• Business model

Methodology of expansion

There are three ways that partners can expand their practices:

1 Open the list to new patients.
2 Bid for a new practice or a tendered practice.
3 Acquire an existing practice.

Opening the list to new patients

Encouraging new patients to join seems straightforward, but the following example illustrates how important it is to ensure the whole practice team understands and shares the partners' vision:

The Crimson practice extended its boundary into an adjacent area and marketed its services with the intention of adding 1,000 patients to the list. The partners were well known and highly respected. As they had expanded their list size in this way in the past, they were surprised when it failed to grow as expected. In an attempt to understand where the barriers to joining lay, one of the partners asked a relative to cold call the practice. His enquiry met with a particularly unwelcoming response from the receptionist, who explained that the GPs were extremely busy and there was already pressure on the patient numbers. She also said any new patient needed to obtain an excessive amount of documentation from the previous practice. Armed with this information, the partners met with all the staff to explain their end aims for the practice and also address the receptionist's concerns that everyone was too busy to take on more patients.

Partners know that each patient attracts approximately £105 from core NHS sources, but receptionists and other staff do not consider this link with the health of the practice. For many partners, simply explaining their aims will engage staff in the process and enable practice growth. In some circumstances it is appropriate to reward staff for helping to attract new patients, or to explain clearly to them exactly when more resources will be brought in to help manage the increased workload.

Marketing to new patients can take many forms:

The Gregory Practice arranged a fun run for the local community on a Sunday morning providing refreshments, prizes and sponsored entertainment. At the end of the run, each participant received a medal, a goody bag with food, drink and a practice registration form.

Rules governing doctors advertising and marketing have always been strict but are more relaxed today than they used to be. Thirty years ago the General Medical Council (GMC) cautioned an East London GP for a photograph appearing in a local newspaper of her standing outside her new surgery. It was considered unacceptable promotional advertising. Today the GMC regulations on advertising as illustrated in the extracts from their Good Medical Practice guidance (Box 6.1) are sensible and protect both patients and doctors.

Box 6.1   Extracts from the GMC regulations on advertising

'If you publish information about your medical services, you must make sure the information is factual and verifiable'.

'You must not make unjustifiable claims about the quality or outcomes of your services in any information you provide to patients. It must not offer guarantees or cures, nor exploit patients' vulnerability or lack of medical knowledge'.

'You must not put pressure on people to use a service, for example by arousing ill-founded fears for their future health'.

Extracts from Good Medical Practice (2006). Reproduced with permission of the General Medical Council.

Bidding for a new practice

Since the 2004 contract was implemented, practices can be run by organisations outside the traditional NHS family, known as Alternative Providers of Medical Services (APMS). This move by the private sector to take over existing practices has encouraged primary care trusts (PCTs) to develop their APMS contracts for financial benefit. A provider with outside business interests may accept a relatively low value contract initially in order to

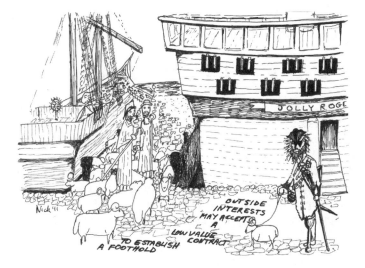

establish a foothold. They will use other resources to finance a loss making business and will not be interested in making a profit at first, because their long term strategy is to acquire practices at their individual value, but sell the accumulated portfolio at a premium.

Using breakeven analysis as a tool

GPs wishing to expand by bidding for a surgery which is being pursued by an external business must ensure their bid is competitive but at the same time sufficiently valuable to their own practice. This involves calculating the minimum funding which makes the contract viable, because APMS providers often accept a much lower price than the average patient value of £105 for core NHS services.

The breakeven analysis is key to reaching a financial, not emotional, decision about contracts.

Costs can be separated into two types; fixed and variable, which relate to the activity in question. Fixed costs do not change with activity, while variable costs do. The following example differentiates the two costs:

A start-up business pays a year's rent in advance of £10,000, and hires a receptionist on £20,000. The business manufactures stethoscopes which retail at £99 each. Each stethoscope takes an hour to make and requires £4 worth of raw materials and a skilled worker at £15 an hour. In this simple case, the fixed costs are the rent and the receptionist's salary. The variable costs are the cost of raw materials and the skilled workers' hourly rate.

This information forms the basis for the following calculations:

$$\text{Selling Price} - \text{Variable Costs} = \text{Net Contribution}$$

$$\frac{\text{Fixed Costs}}{\text{Net Contribution}} = \text{Breakeven Point}$$

In this example, the net contribution is the selling price of £99 minus variable costs £15 + £4, which equals £80.

Fixed costs are £30,000. Therefore the business needs to sell £30,000/£80 = 375 units to break even.

After that point, each stethoscope sold will bring £80 profit, which is the net contribution per stethoscope into the business.

This simple tool is used to calculate the bid value for a new contract.

A typical tender will produce the following information:

Indigo Practice Details
3,000 patients
Existing costs (per annum):

Receptionists	£30,000
Practice manager	£40,000
Nurses	£30,000
Admin and secretarial	£25,000
Rent and rates	Reimbursed by NHS
Heat and light	£6,000
Insurance	£2,000
Drugs and instruments	£4,000
Locum costs	£25,000
Accountancy costs	£5,000

The GPs wishing to bid for the practice will need to decide what price to set for the bid, and to do this they will do the following workings:

Assumptions post take-over

The partners will first need to agree how the practice will function post acquisition and put these assumptions into their plan. Let us assume they agree the following:

• The patient list size will reduce by 500 to 2,500 patients.
• The locum will be replaced by 1.5 salaried GPs costing £120,000 including on-costs.
• All the existing staff will be retained, but nursing costs may rise or fall depending on the number of patients.
• The practice, having taken over the practice, expects to make a profit of £20,000.

Workings

The expenses listed above are then shown as follows:

Receptionists	£30,000	Fixed
Practice manager	£40,000	Fixed
Nurses	£30,000	Variable
Admin and secretarial	£25,000	Fixed
Rent and rates	Reimbursed by NHS	
Heat and light	£6,000	Fixed
Insurance	£2,000	Fixed
Drugs and instruments	£4,000	Variable
Accountancy costs	£5,000	Fixed
Salaried GP costs	£120,000	Fixed
Profit required	£20,000	Fixed

Fixed costs are £248,000.

Variable costs are £30,000 + £4,000 = £34,000.

Variable costs per patient are £34,000/2,500 = £13.60.

Since the breakeven point is

$$\frac{\text{Fixed Costs}}{\text{Net Contribution}}$$

and

$$\text{Net Contribution} = \text{Selling Price} - \text{Variable Costs}$$

if y is the price per patient and 2,500 patients remain, then inserting what is known gives the following:

$$2,500 = \frac{£248,000}{y - £13.60}$$

Simple algebra simplifies this to:

$$2,500y - £34,000 = £248,000$$
$$2,500y = £282,000$$
$$y = £112.80 \text{ per patient}$$

Proof:

Income per patient (£112.80 × 2,500)	£282,000
Less fixed costs	£248,000
Variable costs (£13.60 × 2,500)	£34,000
Surplus (remember, 'profit' is in the fixed costs)	0

If the practice entered a lower bid, it would either receive less profit or make a loss. Sometimes the wish to win the bid can cloud the financial issues and lead the practice to enter a bid that, while being successful, would obligate the practice to provide a level of service that will involve the GPs losing money.

The two approaches to increasing the list by either opening the list or winning a bid will have different consequences for the practice. The first is essentially a slow process, and at certain key intervals the practice will require additional resources. If the list is increasing by 200 patients per quarter, the partners would be unwise to hire a full time salaried GP who will have to wait two years until they reach capacity. It may be preferable to employ locums for the short term until the list has grown sufficiently to take on a part time salaried GP.

Acquiring an existing practice

The third option to expanding a practice is to take over an existing practice. This has financial and longevity advantages over the tendering option:

1 *Financial:* If the practice is put out to tender, the bidding will be competitive and significant weight will be given to the lowest cost. This could possibly outweigh clinical factors.

2 *Longevity:* A typical tendered APMS contract will have a limited life, usually 5 years, after which it will be re-tendered. Existing Personal Medical Services (PMS) or General Medical Services (GMS) contracts are effectively lifetime contracts, and although there has been speculation about changing this, currently a GMS or PMS practice will only be taken away from a GP in catastrophic circumstances.

There are a number of ways an existing GP practice can be acquired, but the following scenario covers many of the issues:

The six-partner Brown practice wished to acquire Dr Black's single-handed surgery.

To achieve this, two of the partners from the Brown practice joined Dr Black's surgery as partners while also retaining their original partnership.

The new three-GP partnership then signed an agreement specifying that Dr Black would retire in 12 months' time.

A year later, Dr Black did indeed retire and his two remaining partners shared the profits with their four original colleagues. This meant the six partners in the Brown practice ended up sharing the profits from both practices equally. After six months had passed, the practice began discussions with the PCT to merge the contracts.

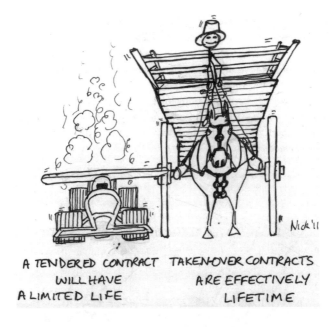

A TENDERED CONTRACT   TAKEN-OVER CONTRACTS
      WILL HAVE   ARE EFFECTIVELY
   A LIMITED LIFE   LIFETIME

What is goodwill?

Goodwill is frequently raised when negotiating the acquisition of a practice or indeed any small business.

Goodwill is the amount of money or money's worth that someone is prepared to pay over and above the value of the assets being acquired. So if a practice has net assets of £100,000 and someone is willing to pay £120,000 for it, the goodwill value is £20,000. Selling and buying goodwill are common with accountancy practices, legal practices and even dental practices, but are virtually prohibited in general practice. Doctors in private practice can sell goodwill in the form of, for example, their practice list. However, the regulations specify that, for NHS GPs, trading in goodwill is a criminal offence. The only exception is selling goodwill for additional and enhanced services. This exception only applies where there are separate contracts for the provision of essential services and of additional and enhanced services. The following real example shows how this can be arranged in practice:

The Windmill Group, a large NHS practice in Solihull, offered to buy the Price practice, a 12,000-patient PMS surgery, and to pay an element of goodwill to the partners. The PCT were supportive, as the Windmill's plans were in line with their own strategic objectives. The Price practice had a single contract with the PCT, so selling goodwill would be unlawful. The PCT agreed to split the Price practice's contract into two: one for the essential services, and another for the additional and enhanced services. The Windmill Group merged with the partners in the Price practice for 12 months, after which the Price partners left. Each leaving partner received nothing from the transfer of the contract to provide essential services, and a five-figure sum for the transfer of the additional and enhanced services. This arrangement only worked because the PCT assisted the contractual changes.

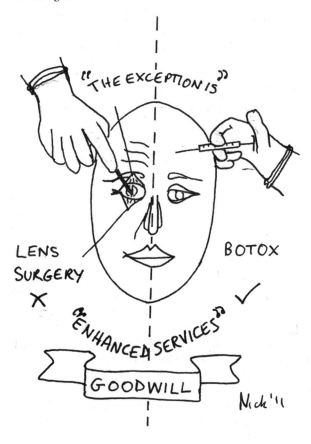

Key points

- Businesses never stand still.
- Beware the risk of over-trading.

- Partnerships can expand by opening their list, bidding for a new or tendered practice or acquiring new practices.
- GPs can market their practice within the guidelines.
- Use breakeven analysis to calculate the value of a new activity.
- Goodwill is money paid over and above the value of the assets acquired.
- For GPs, trading in goodwill can be a criminal act but is possible in certain specified circumstances.

Chapter 7 **Planning for the exit**

Every GP will leave their practice at some stage. This departure may be planned through retirement, or unplanned through such events as expulsion or even death. Preparing for, and managing, the departure is vital to ensure it is smooth and painless.

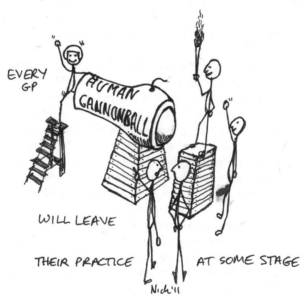

The partnership agreement becomes key in managing exits. The ideal agreement will include details on the following:
1 The notice period for a partner wishing to retire.
2 The terms on which a partner can be expelled.

How to Manage Your GP Practice, First Edition. Farine Clarke and Laurence Slavin.
© 2012 John Wiley & Sons, Ltd. Published 2012 by John Wiley & Sons, Ltd.

3 When a retiring partner should expect to receive their money.

4 How a retiring partner's share is valued.

Partnership disputes are sadly common, and are usually based on disputes over money or workload. Without an agreement, the partnership is technically a partnership at will, as governed by the 1890 Partnership Act, meaning any partner can dissolve it by simply announcing that the partnership is over. As a result:

1 The partnership is immediately dissolved.

2 The bank will freeze the bank account.

3 The outgoing partner is entitled to their funds on the date they leave and on any delay earns interest at 5% on the outstanding balance.

In most practices the partners will have a positive capital or current account balance even in cases where they may not own the premises. These capital or current accounts reflect each partner's financial commitment to the practice which usually ends when that partner leaves. There are exceptions when a partner may leave funds in the practice if, for example, withdrawing them jeopardises the financial position or they wish to maintain an interest in the premises.

Typically a partner in a GP practice will have a balance of £10,000–20,000 in their current account, excluding the premises. The final balance will not be available until the last set of accounts covering the period in which the partner retired have been prepared and agreed by the GPs. Accordingly it is important to allow sufficient time in the partnership agreement for the accounts to be prepared and for subsequent agreement between the partners. Typical arrangements include an obligation to pay after a specified period, often six months post the departure date, or after the final accounts have been agreed. Problems arise with the former if the accounts are delayed due to outstanding information or matters in dispute, and the latter if one or more partner uses the opportunity to delay agreeing the accounts thereby delaying payment to the outgoing partner. The partners need to decide which approach suits them best and ensure this policy is clearly stated in the agreement.

The scenarios under which a partner leaves a practice will bring their own benefits and problems.

The partner voluntarily leaves the practice

This is the most common and least problematic situation, mainly because the leaving and the continuing partners have had time to plan for the departure and are doing so on good terms.

Matters such as replacing the partner and how much they will be repaid are likely to have been carefully discussed and agreed.

The timing and presentation of the practice accounts are vital because these determine the final balance due to the leaving partner.

The partnership agreement usually states that accounts should be drawn up to the date that a partner leaves, even if that date is not the usual year end. This means the practice will have to pay for an extra set of accounts which will cost around 75% of the usual annual charge. Practices occasionally try to save money by requesting one set of accounts and dividing up the profits between the periods when the leaving partner was active and when they left. This can be successful, depending on the attitude of the partners involved. If the partners are unable to take a broad overview of the practice finances and concentrate on the detail, the one extended set of accounts is unlikely to produce an acceptable consensus.

Drs Todd and Patel had been partners for 15 years. The partnership consistently made an annual profit of £300,000 which they shared equally. Their accounting year end was 31 March. Dr Todd retired on 30 September 2010 and was replaced by a salaried GP costing £150,000 per annum.

Clearly in the six month period from March to September, Dr Todd would have a profit share of £75,000, and six-month accounts for that period would demonstrate this. However, annual accounts alone would show the following:

Profits to 31 March 2011	£300,000
Less salaried GP costs (Sept 2010 to Mar 2011)	−75,000
Profits	225,000
Profits shared out as follows	
From 1 April 2010 to 30 September 2010	
Dr Patel share: 50% of £6m profits	56,250
Dr Todd share: 50% of £6m profits	56,250
From 1 October 2010 to 31 March 2011	
Dr Patel share 100% of £6m profits	112,500
Dr Todd share	Nil
Overall profit shares	
Dr Patel	168,750
Dr Todd	56,250
Total	225,000

While it is obvious Dr Todd is due £75,000, the accounts show he is only entitled to £56,250. This is because one set of accounts for the whole period shares all costs and income streams over the year equally. In this case, the salaried GP costs that relate to the period after Dr Todd left have been apportioned over the whole year. Income streams and expenses which are not received or incurred evenly throughout the year should be apportioned to the partners they relate to if one set of accounts is requested to reduce costs. If this is done, the apportionment of profits above would look like this:

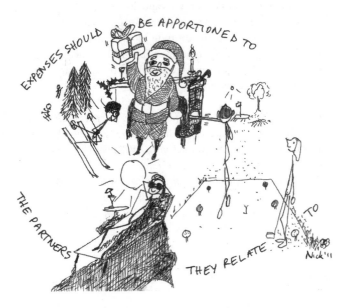

Profits to 31 March 2011	£300,000
Less six months salaried GP costs	−75,000
Profits (as before)	225,000

Profit shares – profits relating to specific partners
Dr Patel bears salaried GP costs post 1 October 2010

Salaried GP costs	− 75,000

Ignoring the salaried GP that has been allocated to Dr Patel, the remaining profits are now £300,000 (i.e. £225,000 + £75,000).

Accordingly,

Profit allocation – to 30 September

Dr Patel share: 50% of £6m profits	75,000
Dr Todd share: 50% of £6m profits	75,000

Profit allocation – to 31 March 2011

Dr Patel share 100% of £6m profits	150,000
Dr Todd share	Nil

Overall profit shares

Dr Patel (£75,000 + £150,000 − £75,000)	150,000
Dr Todd	75,000
Total	225,000

It is highly unlikely that all expenses, such as those for stationery, will be allocated correctly between the periods before and after the partnership change as this is extremely time consuming and costly. Major expenditures such as salaried GP costs should be adjusted for. This means that the use of just one set of accounts only works where there is a positive and amicable approach to apportioning the profits between the two periods. Where the retirement is voluntary and amicable, this approach is usually appropriate.

Involuntary retirement

A partner may leave the practice involuntarily for a variety of reasons. These include being struck off the General Medical Council (GMC) register, breaking a clause in the partnership agreement or falling victim to a 'green socks' clause. The 'green socks' clause is one in which the partners can vote for a colleague to be expelled without having to give a reason, hence the offence of 'wearing green socks'. At the time of writing, there have not been any challenges to this clause under European legislation, although the authors believe that there may be in the future. In such a case, the leaving partner is usually upset, and unlikely to approach the accounts in a positive light. In these cases, it is sensible to prepare two sets of accounts covering the periods before and after the partner leaves.

The extreme example below illustrates what can happen when a partnership agreement fails to address the exit should a newly appointed partner fail their trial period:

The Essex-based Silver practice was a longstanding, well regarded, six-partner surgery. To cope with an increasing workload, the GPs hired Dr Herbert as a partner on an agreed six-month trial period. At the end of this trial, they decided against offering him a permanent post because they were concerned about his competence. The partners informed him of their decision on Friday afternoon, and returned on Monday morning to find Dr Herbert had rearranged the surgery and given himself a consulting room. Dr Herbert accepted that his period of mutual assessment had ended with a termination of his partnership. However, he claimed he had acquired rights to start his own practice from the premises. The partners were forced into a protracted and expensive legal battle. They eventually evicted Dr Herbert but changed all their passkeys and locks as an additional precaution!

The above case highlights the difficulties which ensue when a partnership, however brief, comes to an end with a disgruntled GP. Clearly expecting Dr Herbert to agree the final year-end accounts is unrealistic.

A partner leaving a practice will be owed funds in their capital or current account. It may be prudent not to pay these out until the leaving partner has approved the accounts. This encourages the outgoing partner to reach an agreement over the balances. By contrast, a hostile partner who has received all their funds before approving the accounts has no real motivation to sign off the figures.

For many partnerships, it is sensible to retain a small sum from the leaving partner's capital or current account in the practice to cover any unexpected or unpredicted expenses. Typically this will be up to £5,000.

When a partner leaves involuntarily, the communication between them and the practice is frequently via lawyers and accountants. These professionals will have their clients' interests at heart, not only to ensure the best deal but also to protect themselves from being sued for negligence. Under these circumstances, the practice will wish to retain any commercially sensitive information, so the accounts should only be prepared to the date of the partner's retirement.

Death of a partner

The partnership ends immediately when a partner dies. The continuing partners, who may have had a long and productive relationship with the deceased, will find themselves dealing with family, executors and solicitors. Each of these parties may have differing expectations and competing interests. The partnership agreement, if properly constructed, can come into its own under these circumstances by facilitating the smooth management of the deceased partner's interests in the practice.

Valuing a partner's estate

In the case of a partner's death, it is always worth preparing a new set of accounts to that date including any outstanding income and expenditure. As already stated, goodwill cannot be included in the finances of general practice. The rules are clear, but solicitors frequently bring up goodwill when trying to value a partner's estate. Furthermore, valuing premises can be contentious:

A Bristol practice purchased and extended its surgery three times over a three-year period at a cost of £480,000. The notional rent from the primary care trust (PCT) was £55,000.

Local agents gave the building a bricks and mortar valuation of £500,000 in its current state, but pointed out the premises were in the heart of an area of proposed major redevelopment, which, if this were approved, would raise its value to over £1m.

In the above example, the original costs are irrelevant. The rental income suggests a valuation of £916,000. This is because an external landlord expecting the usual 6% return would pay £916,000 − (6% of £916,000 = £55,000). However any outgoing partner would be aggrieved to be paid their share of £500,000 or £916,000 if the premises sold for £1m a year later.

For reasons such as this, the partnership agreement should specify the basis for valuation. In cases where it does not, the rental value usually takes precedence over the bricks and mortar valuation. In this example, it would be unfair for remaining partners to receive an 11% return on the leaving partner's share.

Development value is more problematic, but the partnership agreement can still include a sliding scale of entitlements if the building is sold post retirement (Table 7.1).

Funding a retiring or deceased partner

When the final accounts are completed, the practice must pay the outgoing partner or their estate. Every partner in every practice will have a balance in

Table 7.1 Sliding renumeration scale for retiring partner

Period between retirement and date of sale	% of development value to be paid to retiring partner
Less than 12 months	100
Between 12 and 18 months	80
Between 18 and 24 months	60
Between 24 and 30 months	40
Between 30 and 36 months	20
After 36 months	Nil

the capital or current account, and the amounts will vary depending on the assets held by the practice on the date the partner leaves.

There are three scenarios for payment:

1 The outgoing partner is paid out of funds saved by the practice.
2 The outgoing partner is paid from a loan raised by the practice.
3 The outgoing partner is paid out of funds introduced by an incoming partner.

1. Paying out of funds saved

This requires the remaining partners to leave funds in the practice.

Dr Adams was retiring from the three-partner Yellow practice. The current accounts were as follows:

Current accounts	Dr Adams	Dr Bott	Dr Caldicott	Total
Balance at 31 March 2010	45,000	15,000	15,000	75,000

If Dr Adams was simply paid his balance, the accounts would show:

Current accounts	Dr Adams	Dr Bott	Dr Caldicott	Total
	0	15,000	15,000	30,000

Clearly this depletes the practice assets and leaves it financially vulnerable. The following scenario would preserve the capital base:

Current accounts	Dr Adams	Dr Bott	Dr Caldicott	Total
	0	37,500	37,500	75,000

To achieve this, Drs Bott and Caldicott would have to either leave a significant part of their profits in the practice or introduce funds into it to pay Dr Adams. Paying a leaving partner out of retained funds means the remaining partners are effectively using profits on which they have already paid tax. This is because tax is paid on the partner's profits, not the income they actually draw. In the above case, the effect for Drs Bott and Caldicott would be as follows:

Dr Bott or Caldicott profit share	£100,000
(after superannuation and expenses)	
Tax thereon	£35,500
After tax profit per GP	£64,500

The retention rate on the £100,000 profit is 64.5%.

If Drs Bott or Caldicott leave an extra £22,500 in their respective current accounts to take them to £37,500, the effect will be as follows:

Dr Bott or Caldicott profit share (after superannuation and expenses)	£100,000
Tax thereon	£35,500
Funds retained in the practice	£22,500
Profit per GP, after tax and retention	£42,000

The retention rate falls dramatically to 42% because the taxation burden has not changed.

For many GPs, paying a partner out of retained funds either is not personally affordable or depletes the practice assets too much, and the partnership elects to borrow the money.

2. Paying a partner out of borrowed funds

The practice bankers usually provide two types of finance to pay an outgoing partner: a loan or an overdraft facility (Figure 7.1).

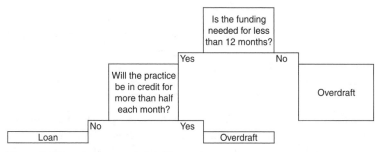

Figure 7.1 Loan versus overdraft facility.

GPs sometimes regard an overdraft as a sign of financial failure which is to be avoided at all costs. However, as a short term solution for cash flow difficulties overdrafts are often appropriate. This is particularly true for practices which experience financial peaks and troughs each month.

In the example above, we can assume the payment to Dr Adams will result in a practice overdraft of £45,000 for two weeks each month. This overdraft will cost £1,350 per annum at an interest rate of 6%. It is eligible for tax relief at say 40% making the actual cost £810, or £405 to each remaining partner. There is also an annual arrangement fee, which is typically 1% or £450 and which is also eligible for tax relief. The £45,000 will have to be repaid eventually, but the overdraft affords the partners flexibility to decide how and when.

The main risk of an overdraft is that it is repayable on demand; the bank can call in the money at any time. Interest rates may also be higher than those on a loan, but interest on a loan is paid throughout the loan period, whereas it is only charged on an overdraft when the account is overdrawn.

3. Paying the outgoing partner from funds introduced by the incoming partner

To assume that an incoming partner pays an outgoing partner on joining a practice is technically incorrect. Responsibility for paying off the leaving partner rests with the partnership, while the new partner buys into the practice with the continuing partners.

In the above example, if Dr Drew replaces Dr Adams and profits are shared with Dr Bott receiving 25%, Dr Caldicott 25% and Dr Drew 50%, the money required to repay Dr Adams and to introduce sufficient funds, by partner, is shown:

	Dr Adams £	Dr Bott £	Dr Caldicott £	Dr Drew £	Total £
Balances at Dr Adams' retirement	45,000	15,000	15,000	0	75,000
Correct balances at Dr Drew's joining	0	18,750	18,750	37,500	75,000
Funds to be withdrawn	45,000	0	0	0	45,000
Funds to be introduced	0	3,750	3,750	37,500	45,000

In this scenario, the partners provide the funds to repay Dr Adams, and the practice does not require a loan. Drs Bott and Caldecott find £3,750 each relatively easily, and in this case Dr Drew has £37,500 from a previous partnership. GPs taking their first partnership post are unlikely to have funds available and are sometimes allowed time to build up their current account balance by drawing less than their profit share each month. It can take five years or so to introduce sums of approximately £40,000 in this way. This is why practices may require a combination of loan, under-drawing and overdraft to manage the reducing debt.

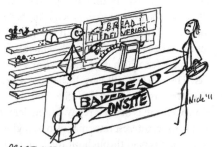

PRACTICES MAY REQUIRE A COMBINATION OF LOAN, UNDERDRAWING & OVERDRAFT

Partner joining with stages to parity

In the 1980s and 1990s, it was common for a three-year discount to be applied to a new partner's profit entitlement. As GPs' profits fell in the early 2000s, the difference between a locum GP's income and a partner's profit share became negligible, meaning practices could not justify imposing this discount. This, coupled with the need to attract the decreasing number of GPs seeking partnerships, meant most new partners joined at full parity. Since the 2004 GP contract, principals are again earning considerably more than locum or salaried GPs, and the concept of parity has returned.

Calculating parity profits

Suppose Dr Schmidt joins a partnership with Drs Burns and Crane under the following terms;

Year 1: 80% of parity

Year 2: 90 % of parity

Year 3: 100% at parity

All partners will have an equal share of profits after three years. There are many methods of calculating parity, but only one is correct and the following mistake is often made:

> In year 1 Dr Schmidt receives a profit share of 26.66% (80% × 1/3). Therefore Drs Burns and Crane receive the balance (i.e. 36.67% each). However, Dr Schmidt is only getting 72.7% of a parity full share (26.66%/36.67%) because the methodology is incorrect.

The correct calculation would apply the discount to Dr Schmidt's share, and calculate new percentages using the discounted rate together with the other partners' share:

	Dr Schmidt	Dr Burns	Dr Crane	Total
Pre-parity shares	33.34%	33.33%	33.33%	100%
80% parity ratios	26.67	33.33	33.33	93.33
80% parity percentages	28.58%	35.71%	35.71%	100%

After adjustment, Dr Schmidt's percentage is now 80% of the other partners' (i.e. 28.58 /35.71).

Another misconception among new partners progressing to full parity is that the reduced parity share will assist in building up their current account. This is only true if the new partner draws less than their profit share. Since the profit share is reduced, there is often no build-up of capital.

Buying in and out of premises

A practice may own its premises separate from its current account. The property owning partners receive rent from the NHS out of which they pay the mortgage, building insurance and other landlord costs. By the time a partner reaches retirement, the mortgage may be partially or fully repaid, and the level of rent will have increased generating rental profits.

At retirement, the partners have three options on the property:

1 Buy out the retiring partner.
2 Allow an incoming partner to buy out the retiring partner's share.
3 Allow the retiring partner to continue to own their share of the premises and receive any profit from the rental.

1. Buy out the retiring partner

This is the most common event. Once the valuation is agreed, the partners usually borrow the funds from their bank or lender to pay the outgoing partner. For tax reasons, timing is critical. This is because there are differential rates for capital gains tax on the sale of a share of a surgery building, with lower rates applied to business assets. This means there are pitfalls in owning the surgery for too long post retirement and losing the business asset relief. It is prudent to divest an interest in the property within a year of retirement. This makes taking professional accountancy advice important for retiring partners.

Once the remaining partners have purchased the retiring partner's share of the property, they will also acquire their share of the rental income, which is used to pay for landlord costs such as the mortgage.

2. Allow an incoming partner to buy the outgoing partner's share of the property

When a new partner buys an outgoing partner's share of the property, the transition is smooth and does not involve the remaining members of the partnership. However, problems arise when the new partner fails their period of mutual assessment but has already bought into the practice. To avoid this, the leaving partner may delay selling their share of the property for the trial period. It is increasingly common for new partners to join practices without buying a share of the property.

3. Allow the retiring partner to continue to own their share of the premises and receive any profit from the rental

This relatively recent development arose in response to practices not replacing partners with new partners and the resulting difficulty in raising finance, together with the uncertainty that notional rents will continue to be paid. The retiring partner effectively becomes an external landlord for their share of the ownership and the practice pays them rental, out of which they fund any mortgage repayments. Partners who take this alternative option should also consider the implications for capital gains tax if the property is not sold at the time of retirement.

Key points

- The partnership agreement is key to managing exits.
- Any partner can effectively dissolve the agreement.
- A typical partner will have £10,000–20,000 in their current account.
- Agree at which point post-departure outstanding payments will be made.
- Exercising the 'green socks clause' is likely to result in an uncooperative leaving partner.
- Dealing with representatives of a deceased partner can be different from the original relationship.
- The partnership agreement should detail how a partner's estate is valued.
- Funding an outgoing partner from practice savings, a loan or the incoming partner has different benefits.

Chapter 8 **Ten questions answered**

Question 1: Why does cash flow matter?

Cash flow is literally the flow of money into and out of a business. At a practical level, cash flow matters because it determines whether or not a business can pay its bills. Those running a business for the first time often have a false sense of security about the viability of their company because they confuse what is owed to them with what is actually in their bank account.

For example, a business which is owed £10k from its clients may feel it can easily pay bills totalling £5k, with £5k to spare. However, if the £10k which is owed has not come in or is delayed, then the company will have to either delay paying its own bills and incur associated penalties, or pay using a bank loan with the accompanying additional charges. In the worst case, the company will fail because its creditors force them into bankruptcy.

Cash flow therefore also involves timing and phasing. Timing of money in and money out is crucial to ensure sufficient funds are in an account when bills are paid. Phasing is another form of 'timing' which accountants and directors use to ensure the cash flow in a business runs effectively and keeps that business in the black rather than the red.

Budgets are usually set months before they go 'live', but circumstances can change; for example, the marketplace may be less buoyant or suppliers may raise costs. For this reason, company directors may 'rephase' their budgets when they are underway to accommodate these changes. This means the monthly accounts will still be compared to a correct, up to date budget, rather than a less realistic one, which in turn means the cash flow of the business will be more accurately monitored.

Companies manage their cash flows in a variety of ways. Some incentivise early payments of money due and penalise late payments. Other, more

How to Manage Your GP Practice, First Edition. Farine Clarke and Laurence Slavin.
© 2012 John Wiley & Sons, Ltd. Published 2012 by John Wiley & Sons, Ltd.

ruthless directors manage their cash flow to their advantage by aggressively claiming payments owed while at the same time withholding payments due for as long as possible.

For many businesses, there is a fine line between encouraging clients to pay on time and penalising them at the risk of damaging the relationship.

Cash flow is not simply an accounting or business concept, but a real entity which determines the viability of a company. Anyone running a business must be on top of their cash flow and able to adapt readily in order to maintain good company health.

Question 2: Why should I understand the accounts? After all, that's what I pay my accountant for.

As a general point, the more you understand your accounts, the greater your understanding of your practice. A keen grasp of the accounts gives you not only an overview of the profit and loss for the practice, but also a feel for the finer details of the business. This matters because the more you understand about the business you run, the greater control you have over it and the more influence you can exert on its progress. Details on the sources of income, the expenses, the ability to pay drawings and whether these should be paid evenly over the year or retained against a potential reduction in profits, as well as the financial requirements of the practice, all become clear. For this reason, view the time you spend with your accountant as an educational opportunity to become more business-minded and gain a deeper understanding of the nuances of your practice.

Most partners see their accountant once a year, and a few see them at more frequent intervals perhaps every six months or even quarterly, but this is a far cry from a company with a finance director who keeps a constant professional eye on the money. During the practice year, partners will make decisions which impact the finances either directly or indirectly and which cannot wait for the accountant visit. Furthermore accountants prepare and report the historical events of the practice, and while they may input into future plans they are not always the best people to advise on daily management. Many accountants have witnessed small businesses fail, making them very cautious when it comes to business decisions.

For these reasons, GP partners in successful practices have a sound understanding of their accounts and use the information to work in partnership with them.

Question 3: What is the point in budgeting – surely the money the practice makes each year is whatever it was going to make?

The financial outcome of a practice is not automatically pre-determined; the partners make informed choices throughout the year which can influence the overall profit and loss.

At a simple level, budgeting is the process of documenting likely income and expenditure each month, reviewing the financial annual outcome and making decisions in advance to influence this.

For instance, if a budget for the year shows a shortfall of £30,000 the partners can plan to mitigate against this. They may decide to try to raise their income by registering a further 350 patients or taking on enhanced services. Or they may try to reduce expenses by limiting staff pay rises, or phasing them to affect only part of the year rather than the full 12 months. Whatever they decide, without a budget the partners would be unaware of the problem and unable to influence the end result.

To prepare and use a budget requires nothing more than a spreadsheet, a knowledge of the past income and expenses, which is available from the practice accounts, an estimate of the future income and expenses based on market intelligence, and an open mind.

The process of preparing a budget in itself focuses everyone's mind on the finances, which in turn benefits the practice. This is similar to the practice of self-monitoring in medicine where patients with conditions such as diabetes gain awareness of their condition by regularly testing their blood glucose levels. Simply knowing their numbers helps them to comply with medication and improve their health. In businesses, knowing your numbers gives you more control and power and improves your financial health. As such, budgeting is an invaluable tool for anyone involved in running any type of business.

Question 4: I am joining a partnership, and have been told that I need to pay in £5,000 for my share of the assets. Why don't we treat the assets as having no value, so no one needs to leave any money in the practice?

This question touches on a number of issues affecting GPs. When a partner joins a practice, they are joining as a co-owner. Ensuring the practice has sufficient resources to function is one of the responsibilities of co-ownership. The partners' capital or current accounts added together equal the net assets in the practice. A partner who earns more profits than they draw from the practice will leave funds in the bank and also increase their capital or current account. If the capital accounts had no value, the practice would have no assets. This is rarely the case as practices have assets such as equipment and money in the bank to cover the day to day running costs. Creating a practice with nil assets is engineered occasionally by taking sufficient loans and overdrafts, but it is not recommended.

Ownership of, and responsibility to provide, these assets should be shared fairly between the partners. For example, four GP partners in a practice with net assets of £20,000 will have invested £5,000 each. If one partner leaves taking their £5,000, the three remaining GPs will make up the difference and invest £6,666 in the practice. This means when the new fourth partner joins and invests £5,000, the other partners can withdraw their £1,666 taking everyone's share to the same value.

Valuing the assets can be difficult. While assets with intrinsic values such as the bank balance and debtors and creditors are straightforward, those such as equipment, fixtures, fittings and computers are less specific. They may be valued at a sale value, a replacement value, an insurance value, a net book value or any other method derived by the parties concerned. This makes it important for the value method employed to be transparent and agreed upon in advance. It is prudent for an incoming partner to check the list of practice assets, as there are rare examples of inappropriate inclusions, in one case this took the form of a senior partner's personal Jaguar XJS!

Assets bought with grants or savings from activities in the NHS can be valued either with or without the benefit of the grants. For example, if a practice partially offset £25,000 worth of fixtures, fittings and equipment with £10,000 of activity savings, it only paid £15,000 for the assets. The practice can ask a new partner to buy into these assets at either £25,000 or £15,000 as long as it makes the basis clear.

Buying in can take many forms, from the incoming partner borrowing the money and lending it to the practice or by leaving a small amount of profits in the practice over a number of years. Any method is acceptable if it can be agreed by all the parties.

Question 5: It seems unprofessional and greedy to bill patients within two weeks of a consultation; shouldn't I delay a month or two before sending a bill?

It is not unprofessional to charge patients in a timely fashion following a consultation for which they are expecting to pay. Indeed. it could be argued that doing so shows that you are well organised and efficient, which in turn reflects well on all your abilities and your practice.

Patients, like all of us, do not like inconsistency, but this is particularly true with healthcare where there are other associated anxieties. Therefore it is worth putting down good boundaries as well as a consistent approach by billing your patients within the same timeframe after each consultation. Ensuring your practice has the right systems in place to bill patients and insurance companies quickly and accurately will also minimise errors, save time and money and reduce stress in the long run.

As with any business, the longer the delay in receiving payment for a bill, the more likely that the bill will move from 'late payment' to 'bad debt'. By the time a bill is in the bad debt category, it is less likely to ever be paid. For doctors this means a private consultation becomes a free consultation, unless they are willing to chase that debt. This in turn costs time and money, not to mention the emotional stress and concerns that accompany pursuing a patient. For understandable reasons, many doctors give up on unpaid bills by this stage. It is fair to say that a private consultation is a service for which the professional expects to charge and the client expects to pay. Therefore doctors should feel unapologetic for requesting payment in the same way that any similar professional, be they a lawyer or a dentist, would.

Discomfort is sometimes felt on both sides when an NHS patient does not expect to pay for non-NHS services, such as signing passport applications. In this circumstance it helps to have a system in place which manages expectations. Briefing the receptionists about charges means they can warn patients before the consultation and request payment afterwards.

Charging in an accurate, consistent and timely manner is another example of best practice which minimises errors and debt and is vital to the health of your business.

Question 6: I trust my staff and we have a good relationship, so why do I need to put systems in place to manage them?

The best practices, like the best businesses, will have a happy workforce with a high degree of trust and respect between staff and managers. The ethos of a company, be that nurturing or ruthless, trusting or suspicious, usually derives from the approach of the person or people in charge.

Relationships between staff in the work environment are complex and, while there may be long periods of stability, they are also subject to change depending on what is happening within the business or in the personal lives of its partners or staff.

While trust is a hugely valuable commodity, it is not always sufficient to protect a business or its employees from the vagaries of change. When things become difficult, be that with a member of staff or a fellow partner, it is immensely helpful to have processes in place which both parties understand and can follow. Such processes will bypass any personal or emotive issues and achieve what is best for everyone.

A high level of trust and a robust staff management system are not mutually exclusive within the same practice. Staff do not feel betrayed by managers who put fair systems in place and follow them. Indeed, all good management systems do as much to protect employees as they do the employers. If followed properly, they will also pre-empt potential problems, for example a member of staff may only admit they are running into difficulties at an appraisal meeting with their manager.

Management styles vary hugely amongst GPs, and while this is inevitable, it can expose them to claims of favouritism or bullying. Good systems will ensure a consistent approach to staff issues and mean that whichever partner is involved, the same process will be followed with the same results for the practice. The reassurance which comes with this consistency cannot be over-stated. Staff, particularly in close working environments, feel comfortable knowing that they will be treated the same by each partner and, equally importantly, that their colleagues will be treated exactly the same in the same situation. Partners will be reassured that their peers will treat staff the same, leaving little room for manipulation and division. The effect of all of this is that the practice team functions more smoothly.

As with any system with the potential to be misinterpreted in the workplace, communication is key. Make sure staff understand which systems are in place, why they are there and what they are designed to achieve. The staff handbook is the best place to bring all management issues together so that staff and employers have one reliable point of reference which sets the employment standards for the whole practice.

Good management fulfils a hugely positive role in any business. A management system which includes appraisals, mentoring, professional development and other positive aspects of working life will help employees to progress. Some of the best employers understand the value of good management systems because they were managed very well by others in their own early careers. Everyone appreciates being well managed at work.

Question 7: If a patient or service has not paid me, how can I claim that debt?

In an ideal world, your approach to chasing debt should be the same whether it is from a patient with whom you have a caring relationship, or from a service where your relationship is entirely business focused. However, the doctor–patient relationship is multifaceted, and it is understandable that a GP or private practitioner will approach a patient debt very differently from that owed by a commercial organisation. This is also true in wider business where client trust has been built over several years but can be destroyed in moments. This is why business people will chase debt from a valued client

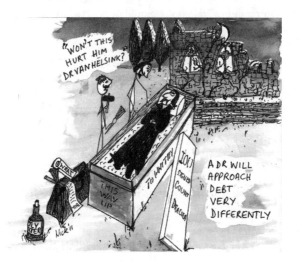

very differently from that owed by a faceless organisation. At the very least, they will have a conversation directly with the client and try to resolve any payment issues rather than allow the finance department to send a routine final demand notice.

An explanation of how late payments can easily become 'bad debt' was given in the previous answer. Determining at what stage a late payment is labelled a bad debt will depend on the type of business and its relationships with its suppliers, services and clients. For many businesses, payment within 30 days of an invoice is the norm. If the money has not been received within three to six months, it may then become a 'bad debt'. If the money is never paid, it may be written off after a year, or sometimes two years.

Some organisations hire people into their finance department specifically to chase any outstanding bad debt towards the end of the accounting year. These individuals will spend the whole working day on the phone requesting payment from late payers. Companies find a percentage of their debt will be recalled by this method and avoid court.

Whatever your approach to late payment, it is worth having a robust system in place to deal with it. The system will identify outstanding debts after a certain date and issue a reminder letter. This may be followed by a second reminder a month later. At any stage the doctor or the doctor's secretary may prefer to try to speak with the patient directly to understand why payment has not been sent.

Taking legal action against patients needs to be decided on an individual basis, but small fees can be claimed through the small claims court while larger amounts may require the help of a solicitor. Claims against the primary care trust (PCT) or another NHS body should be referred to the NHS Litigation Authority in Harrogate.

Chasing debt is expensive, time consuming and stressful which is why it is prudent to have systems in place to receive prompt payments. It is also worth trying to resolve any outstanding debt issues quickly to avoid costly and unpleasant litigation. When the debt is associated with ongoing work, such as writing solicitors or insurance reports, it may be worth ensuring they are paid before agreeing to proceed. All those involved in running small businesses appreciate that bad debt has a negative impact on cash flow which in turn will have a deleterious effect on their company.

Question 8: If my practice grows, won't I automatically make more money?

Just because a business grows in size, or even in revenue, that does not automatically mean its profits will grow in parallel. Indeed, in the early stages of growth, the profits of a company can go down despite the fact that turnover has increased, as money is invested into consolidating and reorganising the business for the aimed for growth ahead.

Small business owners often mistakenly believe that if they grow in scale, and increase their turnover, they will automatically raise their profits. Sadly there are countless examples of companies which overstretched themselves as they expanded and subsequently failed. The stretch reflects lack of expertise at many levels, be they staff or business processes.

At a simple level, keeping abreast of the financial details of a small practice is relatively easy. Fewer patients and staff means there is less of everything to manage, and more time for GP partners to resolve day to day issues. Routine matters like patient claims and outstanding fees are readily dealt with. It is also easier to identify and respond quickly to errors in payments or a sudden increase in the expenses.

As a practice grows, it becomes more complex and the volume of data, staff and patients to deal with increases. There is often a stage in business growth when the workload and revenue have increased significantly but the systems and/or staff is not yet in place to manage these. It is extremely difficult to increase the resources necessary to cope with growth in parallel with the growth itself. Staff recruitment and training alone can account for a delay between the two. Furthermore, businesses are often wary of recruiting new staff in preparation for growth, as this puts a negative pressure on the salary bill until the increased revenues come through.

Maximising income is therefore more difficult in a growing practice as GP partners may find they lose control in the move from a tight claiming small practice to a looser claiming larger one. As the pressure on senior staff grows, financial activities may be delegated to staff lower down the ladder who either lack expertise about the processes or do not view claiming monies as vital to the health of the practice. In extreme circumstances a practice may stop claiming for an entire set of services, and the error is only detected at the compilation of the annual accounts by which time it is too late to collect.

Cost control through growth periods can be very difficult. Planned-for costs as part of a growth strategy are one thing, but unplanned-for costs can frequently appear as a business expands and throw a company off course. For this reason, many businesses put a 'contingency' sum with no specific cause into their growth budgets. This does not reflect an inability to budget correctly, but rather an intrinsic understanding that there will be hidden costs in an expanding business, and while one might not know exactly what they will be, it is preferable to prepare for them than to simply hope they do not occur.

When a GP practice grows in size, either through acquiring a new surgery or by taking on additional patients, it is advisable to compile a growth budget. Working to a plan enables any business to run more smoothly. One of the commonest demands partners face through a growth period is for more staff. If GPs know in advance at which point they will increase staff numbers to cope with increased pressures on the practice, they can communicate this to existing staff in advance. Such explanation will not only allay staff fears but also help them to feel part of the growth strategy and know there is an end point to their increased workload.

Question 9: Surely marketing only applies in the commercial sector, and there's no need to market a GP practice?

In many commercial organisations the marketing director is as important as the managing director or chief executive. This is because marketing is vital to business, but not just commercial ones; any person or service which needs to attract purchasers or end users needs to be able to market to them.

Marketing encompasses a range of disciplines from advertising to PR to word of mouth. As a result it takes many forms at hugely differing costs. The price of a major advertising campaign in a national newspaper is clearly different from that of a few flyers in a local magazine or a round-table meeting to discuss a product. Large commercial organisations have marketing departments staffed by marketers with differing but complementary expertise, whose job it is to ensure the company's products or services are advertised and taken up by the right target groups.

While GP partners may not consider it necessary to market their practice as commercial organisations do, they may still wish to attract new patients or ensure services are taken up. Devising a 'marketing strategy', however small, to achieve this will still be useful. Once partners have focussed on the end aim, they can compile a marketing plan together with details such as who will execute it together with associated costs. Doing this makes the plan more likely to be acted on and less likely to remain on the practice's 'One day we would like to . . .' list.

Of course, as community based surgeries GPs and their staff market the practice every time they see a patient, or refer to a consultant or other health professional. This is one reason why some practices have better reputations than others.

As the NHS continues to undergo relentless change, it may become increasingly useful to market the positive aspects of a practice, not only to local patients, but also to a wide reach of organisations. Building up some marketing expertise will stand any GP practice or partner in good stead.

Question 10: Why do one in three new businesses fail?

It is a sad fact that about a third of new businesses in the United Kingdom fail within the first five years of launch.

General practice is a relatively secure environment and partners are largely protected compared to wholly commercial directors, but some of the principles which cause new businesses to fail can also damage a GP practice.

1 *Cash flow*: Late payments and resultant inability to pay bills are frequently cited as the commonest reasons for a small business to fail. We have already discussed at length the need to ensure that money flows into and out of a business in a manner which keeps it viable, and prevents debtors from fore-closing the company. Many small businesses now include incentives for early payment and penalties for delays as a part of their terms and conditions of service, although extracting payment from late payers who eventually become 'bad debt' is likely to always be a problem.

2 *Misguided or no research*: It is easy for any business owner to be so excited by their new venture and the opportunity to run their own company that they become immune to any evidence against it. This is why it is essential to do research to support any business idea. It is true that not all business successes were founded through focus groups, which in themselves can be self-selecting and flawed, but it is worth sense checking any idea by talking to the target market or looking at the success of similar products. Information, including market data and competitive data, is vital when positioning any new business.

3 *Excessive debt*: Funding a new business can be problematic. Many new businesses are self-funded, which puts excessive strain on the directors. Banks and financial institutions will lend to new businesses, but their flexibility will depend on the economic climate and we have already highlighted examples in general practice where they have called in the debts to the demise of the partners. Ensuring the business is not burdened with too much debt at the outset is key to success.

4 *Expertise*: Having the right number of staff with the right level of expertise may seem obvious, but it is amazing how many business people say that achieving this is extremely difficult if not impossible. Expertise and management skills per se are not the only issues; managing staff morale, turnover and absence through illness can also put tremendous strains on a new business.

5 *Being self-employed*: Founders of new businesses are often very enthusiastic, but they can easily underestimate how difficult it is to stay focused when working alone. Being one's own boss is the dream for many, but without the boundaries of an office, senior management and peers, the

work ethic can be severely dented. Successful entrepreneurs are self-motivated to an extreme. They do not automatically expect to start work at 9 and finish at 5 with an hour for lunch. This does not mean they have the gold standard work–life balance by any means, but the work required to successfully launch a new business is often much greater than most people think.

Chapter 9 **Thou shalt . . . thou shalt not!**

Thou shalt . . .

- Make 'Put the Practice First' your mantra in all management and business decisions.
- Make sure the type of partnership agreement you sign is the right one for your needs.
- Make sure you fully understand the accounts before signing them.
- View money as a vital commodity to keep the practice healthy.
- Put aside protected time for your personal and professional development without feeling guilty.
- Give all employees an up to date staff handbook detailing your practice processes and procedures.
- Protect the boundaries between yourself and your staff, even if you feel disingenuous, for the good of everyone.
- Link your expansion plans to the vision shared between all the partners.
- Ensure practice staff understand and have signed up to your future visions.
- Make provisions for a smooth and painless departure from the partnership.

Thou shalt not . . .

- Practice without agreeing and signing a comprehensive partnership agreement.
- Join a partnership without analysing their accounts.
- Fail to put aside monthly income for tax.
- Fail to put aside dilapidations funds on leased premises.
- Delay invoicing for funds which are owed to you.
- Put yourself or your practice at risk of a discrimination claim from existing or potential staff.

How to Manage Your GP Practice, First Edition. Farine Clarke and Laurence Slavin.
© 2012 John Wiley & Sons, Ltd. Published 2012 by John Wiley & Sons, Ltd.

- Mistake budgeting for a paper exercise.
- Underestimate the importance of cash flow.
- Confuse an ability to manage complex patient problems with an ability to manage simple staff issues.
- Grow the practice without compiling a workable post-acquisition consolidation plan for the expanded business.

Appendix 1: Useful contacts

ACAS: 08457 474747. www.acas.org.uk

BMA: 0207 387 4499. www.bma.org.uk

Federation of Small Businesses: 01253 336000. www.fsb.org.uk

GMC: 0161 923 6602. www.gmc-uk.org

Institute of Chartered Accountants in England and Wales: 01908 248250. www.icaew.com

Institute of Directors: 0207 766 8855. www.iod.com

The Law Society: 0207 242 1222. www.lawsociety.org,uk

RCGP: 0203 188 7400. www.rcgp.org.uk

Royal Institution of Chartered Surveyors: 020 7334 3811. www.rics.org

How to Manage Your GP Practice, First Edition. Farine Clarke and Laurence Slavin.
© 2012 John Wiley & Sons, Ltd. Published 2012 by John Wiley & Sons, Ltd.

Appendix 2: Full set of practice accounts

SUNNIHILL HEALTH CENTRE
ACCOUNTS
FOR THE YEAR ENDED
31 MARCH 2010

PRACTICE INFORMATION

PARTNERS:	Dr Ghode
	Dr Stern
	Dr Hart
SURGERY ADDRESS:	Health Centre
	170 Replay Road
	Chichester
	West Sussex
ACCOUNTANTS:	Davison and Sons
	Chartered Accountants
	Deer House
	8 Lyme Avenue
	Midhurst
	West Sussex
CLIENT REFERENCE:	

How to Manage Your GP Practice, First Edition. Farine Clarke and Laurence Slavin.
© 2012 John Wiley & Sons, Ltd. Published 2012 by John Wiley & Sons, Ltd.

SUNNIHILL HEALTH CENTRE
ACCOUNTS
FOR THE YEAR ENDED
31 MARCH 2010

CONTENTS

	PAGE
Accountants' Report	1
Partners' Certificate	2
Profit and Loss Account	3
Balance Sheet	4
Schedules of Income	5–7
Notes to the Accounts	8–10

SUNNIHILL HEALTH CENTRE
ACCOUNTS
FOR THE YEAR ENDED
31 MARCH 2010

ACCOUNTANTS' REPORT TO THE PARTNERS
OF HEALTH CENTRE
ON THE UNAUDITED ACCOUNTS

We have compiled the accounts of your practice which comprise a profit and loss account, a balance sheet and related notes from the accounting records and information and explanations given to us.

The accounts are not intended to achieve full compliance with the provisions of UK Generally Accepted Accounting Principles.

Our work has been undertaken so that we might compile the accounts that we have been engaged to compile, report to you that we have done so and state those matters that we have agreed to state to you in this report and for no other purpose. To the fullest extent permitted by law, we do not accept or assume responsibility to anyone other than to you for our work, or for this report.

We have carried out this engagement in accordance with technical guidance issued by the Institute of Chartered Accountants in England & Wales and have complied with the ethical guidance laid down by the Institute.

You have approved the accounts for the year ended 31 March 2010 and have acknowledged your responsibility for them, for the appropriateness of the accounting basis and for providing all information and explanations necessary for their compilation.

We have not verified the accuracy or completeness of the accounting records or information and explanations you have given to us and we do not, therefore, express any opinion on the financial information.

Signed:
Date:

2

SUNNIHILL HEALTH CENTRE
ACCOUNTS
FOR THE YEAR ENDED
31 MARCH 2010

PARTNERS' CERTIFICATE

We certify that, to the best of our knowledge and belief, the accounting records provided, together with the information and explanations given to Davison and Sons, constitute a true and correct record of the transactions of our practice for the year ended 31 March 2010, and we confirm that the accounts have our approval.

....
Dr. Ghode

....
Dr. Stern

....
Dr. Hart

Dated 2010

3

SUNNIHILL HEALTH CENTRE
PROFIT AND LOSS ACCOUNT
FOR THE YEAR ENDED 31 MARCH 2010

	Sch £	2010 £	2009 £	£
Fees Earned (Before deduction of £41,699 Superannuation)	1	568,867		549,097
Reimbursements	2	65,305		44,082
Other Income	3	16,606		12,101
		650,778		605,280

LESS OVERHEADS

Salaries and Wages	173,112		150,652
Note Summarising	6,506		5,270
Salaried Assistant	121,498		68,684
Staff Welfare	3,157		3,701
Staff Pension	6,787		5,784
Staff Training	26		1,140
Locums	26,004		17,863
Deputising and Co-op Service	1,917		1,066
Drugs	17,722		13,643
Telephone	6,557		5,119
Computer Expenses	1,580		6,273
Printing, Postage and Stationery	8,068		6,749
Subscriptions	999		1,719
General Expenses	147		151
Hire of Equipment	516		473
Courses and Conferences	424		(126)
Advertising	869		361
Travelling	184		207
Repairs and Maintenance	2,589		700
Insurance	1,150		969
Rent and Rates	24,480		24,000
Parking Permit Charge	2,315		2,920
Health Centre Charges	(607)		10,782
Levies	3,507		2,782
Bank Interest and Charges	914		239
Legal and Professional Fees	3,612		1,533
Accountancy	4,700		4,477
Depreciation	558		656
		(419,291)	(337,787)
NET PROFIT FOR THE YEAR (NOTE 1)		231,487	267,493

4

SUNNIHILL HEALTH CENTRE
BALANCE SHEET
AS AT 31 MARCH 2010

	Note £	2010 £	2009 £	£
FIXED ASSETS				
Tangible Assets	2		3,162	3,720
CURRENT ASSETS				
Stock of Drugs		2,330		2,330
Sundry Debtors and Prepayments		61,682		63,741
Main Bank Account		37,893		48,902
Building Society Account		1,619		21,855
Cash in Hand		1,350		396
		104,874		137,224
CURRENT LIABILITIES				
Taxation		33,116		38,237
Superannuation		7,414		5,476
Sundry Creditors and Accruals		5,634		17,820
		46,164		61,533
NET CURRENT ASSETS		58,710	75,691	
		61,872	79,411	
REPRESENTED BY:				
CURRENT ACCOUNTS	3			
Dr. Ghode		25,304	27,580	
Dr. Stern		21,856	33,866	
Dr. Hart		14,712	17,965	
		61,872	79,411	

5

SUNNIHILL HEALTH CENTRE
SCHEDULES OF INCOME
FOR THE YEAR ENDED 31 MARCH 2010

	Sch	2010 £	2009 £
SCHEDULE 1			
Fees Earned			
Global Sum		341,241	329,254
Staff		–	1,000
Less: Opt-out Out of Hours		(20,206)	(20,973)
Correction Factor		80,910	91,637
Seniority		9,581	8,394
		411,526	409,312
Quality and Outcome Framework	4	112,096	99,767
Enhanced Services	5	45,245	40,018
		568,867	549,097
Registered List		6,255	6,481
Weighted List		5,884	6,097
SCHEDULE 2			
Reimbursements			
Locums		21,187	(533)
Rent and Rates		24,480	24,000
Computer Expenses		–	4,848
Drugs		19,638	15,767
		65,305	44,082

6

SUNNIHILL HEALTH CENTRE
SCHEDULES OF INCOME
FOR THE YEAR ENDED 31 MARCH 2010

	2010 £	2009 £
SCHEDULE 3		
Other Income		
Superannuable		
Student Doctor Training	2,198	–
Non-Superannuable		
Private Fees	12,790	11,236
Bank Deposit Interest	1,618	865
	16,606	12,101

SCHEDULE 4

Quality and Outcome Framework

	2010		Maximum	2009	
	Total £	Number of points	Points Available	Total £	Number of points
Clinical Domain	68,463	653	655	62,514	646
Organisational	21,122	160	181	16,797	140
Additional Services	5,584	36	36	5,025	36
Patient Experience	14,283	108	108	12,919	108
Holistic Care	2,644	20	20	2,512	19
	112,096	977	1,000	99,767	949

7

SUNNIHILL HEALTH CENTRE
SCHEDULES OF INCOME
FOR THE YEAR ENDED 31 MARCH 2010

	2010 £	2009 £
SCHEDULE 5		
Enhanced Services		
Directed Enhanced Services		
Improved Access Scheme	11,083	6,127
Childhood Immunisation Targets	5,241	10,495
Influenza	5,337	6,089
Minor Surgery	362	1,556
Phlebotomy	1,298	748
Information Management and Technology	(37)	2,635
Choose and Book	5,387	–
Post-Operative Care	1,380	2,741
National Enhanced Services		
IUCD Fitting	2,073	2,648
Drug Misuse	813	800
Smoking Cessation	–	965
Local Enhanced Services		
Practice Based Commissioning	11,385	5,214
Methotrexate	563	–
SMEP	360	–
	45,245	40,018

8

SUNNIHILL HEALTH CENTRE
NOTES TO THE ACCOUNTS
FOR THE YEAR ENDED 31 MARCH 2010

1. ALLOCATION OF PROFIT

	Dr. G. £	Dr. S. £	Dr. H. £	Total £
Prior Allocation				
Seniority	6,926	1,969	686	9,581
Balance				
33.30: 44.40: 22.30	73,895	98,526	49,485	221,906
	80,821	100,495	50,171	231,487

9

SUNNIHILL HEALTH CENTRE
NOTES TO THE ACCOUNTS
FOR THE YEAR ENDED 31 MARCH 2010

3. CURRENT ACCOUNTS

	Dr. G. £	Dr. S. £	Dr. H. £	Total £
Balance at 1 April 2009	27,580	33,866	17,965	79,411
Share of Profit	80,821	100,495	50,171	231,487
	108,401	134,361	68,136	310,898
Less:				
Drawings	45,500	53,800	31,560	130,860
Superannuation	13,775	21,475	8,033	43,283
Taxation	23,822	37,230	13,831	74,883
	83,097	112,505	53,424	249,026
Balance at 31 March 2010	25,304	21,856	14,712	61,872

SUNNIHILL HEALTH CENTRE
SCHEDULE OF DRAWINGS
FOR THE YEAR ENDED 31 MARCH 2010

	Dr. G. £	Dr. S. £	Dr. H. £	Total £
MONTH				
April	3,250	3,900	2,300	9,450
May	3,250	3,900	2,300	9,450
June	3,600	4,100	2,500	10,200
July	3,600	4,100	2,500	10,200
August	3,600	4,100	2,500	10,200
September	3,600	4,100	2,500	10,200
October	3,600	4,100	2,500	10,200
November	3,600	4,100	2,500	10,200
December	3,600	4,200	2,500	10,300
January	1,800	2,100	1,250	5,150
February	1,800	2,100	1,250	5,150
March	1,800	2,100	1,250	5,150
	37,100	42,900	25,850	105,850
Additional Drawings	8,400	10,900	5,710	25,010
	45,500	53,800	31,560	130,860

11

SUNNIHILL HEALTH CENTRE
FOR THE YEAR ENDED 31 MARCH 2010
PRACTICE STATISTICS

	Ramsay Brown Guide	2010	2009
Staff Wages Efficiency Ratio	33.00%	$\frac{189,588}{568,867} = 33.33\%$	$\frac{166,547}{549,097} = 30.33\%$
Clinical Assistance Ratio	14.00%	$\frac{128,232}{568,867} = 22.54\%$	$\frac{88,146}{549,097} = 16.05\%$
Administrative Ratio	7.56%	$\frac{28,464}{568,867} = 5.00\%$	$\frac{33,294}{549,097} = 6.06\%$
Financial and Professional Ratio	1.75%	$\frac{9,226}{568,867} = 1.62\%$	$\frac{6,249}{549,097} = 1.14\%$
New Contract Income per Patient Ratio	£110.00	$\frac{568,867}{6,255} = £90.95$	$\frac{549,097}{5,775} = £95.08$
Global Sum Equivalent plus Seniority	£79.00	$\frac{411,526}{6,255} = £65.79$	$\frac{408,312}{5,775} = £70.70$
Quality and Outcome Framework Income	£18.00	$\frac{112,096}{6,255} = £17.92$	$\frac{99,767}{5,775} = £17.28$
Enhanced Services Income	£12.50	$\frac{45,245}{6,255} = £7.23$	$\frac{40,018}{5,775} = £6.93$
Other Income per Patient Ratio	£9.00	$\frac{16,606}{6,255} = £2.65$	$\frac{12,101}{5,775} = £2.10$
Net Profit per Patient Ratio	£55.00	$\frac{231,487}{6,255} = £37.01$	$\frac{267,493}{5,775} = £46.32$
Net Profit per Partner	£133,500	$\frac{231,487}{2.25} = £102,833$	$\frac{267,493}{2.25} = £118,885$

12

SUNNIHILL HEALTH CENTRE
FOR THE YEAR ENDED 31 MARCH 2010
PRACTICE STATISTICS WORKINGS

	2010 £	2009 £
Staff Wages Efficiency Ratio		
Salaries and Wages	173,112	150,652
Note Summarising	6,506	5,270
Staff Welfare	3,157	3,701
Staff Pension	6,787	5,784
Staff Training	26	1,140
	189,588	166,547
Clinical Assistance Ratio		
Salaried Assistant (Net)	101,462	68,684
Locums (Net)	24,853	18,396
Deputising and Co-op Service	1,917	1,066
	128,232	88,146
Administrative Ratio		
Health Centre Charges	–	10,782
Telephone	6,557	5,119
Computer Expenses (Net)	1,580	1,425
Printing, Postage and Stationery	8,068	6,749
General Expenses	147	151
Hire of Equipment	516	473
Courses and Conferences	424	–
Advertising	869	361
Travelling	184	207
Repairs and Maintenance	2,589	700
Insurance	1,150	969
Parking Permit Change	2,315	2,920
Levies	3,507	2,782
Depreciation – Medical Equipment	316	371
Depreciation – Fixtures and Fittings	242	285
	28,464	33,294
Financial and Professional Ratio		
Bank Interest and Charges	914	239
Legal and Professional Fees	3,612	1,533
Accountancy	4,700	4,477
	9,226	6,249

Index

accountancy costs 40, 92, 93
accountants 113–15
    and accounting 37–45, 47, 52, 57, 66,
        69, 71
    and budgeting 74, 79
    and business as organism 1, 2,
        8, 14
    and operational model 83
    and planning for exit 104
    qualifications 45
    report 45
    and staff 18, 19, 30
accounting 37–72
    best system for your practice
        39–41
    software packages 40
accounts
    demystifying 37–9
    importance of understanding 114–15,
        125
    practice (full set) 130–43
acquiring existing practice 94–5
administrative expenses ratio 62, 64, 67
advertising 48, 62, 64, 66, 122, 134, 143
    GMC regulations on 90
allocation of profit 56, 57
annual salary review 26
annual staff appraisal 26
APMS (Alternative Providers of Medical
        Services) 65, 90

appreciating staff 27
Articles Association 7
assets 37
    current 50
    fixed 50
    why pay into 116–17

balance sheets 39, 50–1, 69,
        86
balanced skills 21
best practice staff management
        35
billing patients speedily 117–18
bookkeeping 37, 39, 41, 71
boundaries between GP and staff,
        protecting 125
breakeven analysis 91–4
budgeting 73–9
    and good business practice
        76–9
    importance of 115–16, 126
business
    growth 87–97
        and profit 121–2
    as organism 1–16
buying in and out of premises
        110–11
    allow incoming partner to buy
        outgoing partner's share 110
    buy out retiring partner 110

How to Manage Your GP Practice, First Edition. Farine Clarke and Laurence Slavin.
© 2012 John Wiley & Sons, Ltd. Published 2012 by John Wiley & Sons, Ltd.

buying or renting premises 12–15, 16
　pros and cons 13

candidates for interview, selection of 21–2
capital 37
　accounts 68–70
cash flow 16
　forecasts 79
　importance of 113–14, 126
　problems, as reason for business
　　failure 123
CGT (capital gains tax) 15, 16
claiming debt from non-paying patients
　119–20
cleaning costs 41
clinical assistance ratio 62, 63, 67
Companies Act 83
Companies House 82
competition, practice as being in 15–16
Comprehensive Partnership Agreement
　125
current accounts 58, 68–70
　differential, problems with 70
　and drawings 60
current assets 50, 69
current liabilities 50, 69
CVs 21

death of partner 104–5
　valuing estate 104–5
debts
　as cause of business failure 123
　claiming from non-paying patients
　　119–20
　and obligations, liability for 81–2
decision making, as key to success 4, 7–9, 16
delegation 17
differential current accounts, problems
　with 70
dilapidation funds 125
direct enhanced services 55
direction, as key to success 4, 6–7, 16
disciplinary procedures 33–5
discipline, staff 32–5

discrimination 19
　claims 125
disputes, partnership 100
dividends 84
double entry bookkeeping 40, 41–68
drug(s)
　addiction 30
　theft of 30

earnings, GPs' 88
electricity costs 41
employment law 17–18
enhanced services 55
　income ratio 65
Excel spreadsheet 40
expansion 88–9
　methodology of 89
　plan 89, 125
　see also business growth
expenses 5, 14, 37–40, 47, 49, 57, 63, 68,
　74, 85, 102, 104, 115, 121
　administrative expenses ratio 62, 64,
　　67
expertise, lack of, as cause of business
　　failure 123–4

failure of new businesses, reasons for
　123–4
fees earned 53
financial and professional ratio 62, 64, 67
fixed assets 50, 51, 69, 71, 85
fixed vs variable costs 79
FTE (full time equivalent) partners 49
funding retiring or deceased partner 104,
　105–9
　from borrowed funds 107
　from funds of incoming partner 108–9
　from funds saved 106–7
future visions, staff understanding your
　125

global sum equivalent/baseline, plus
　seniority 65
GMC (General Medical Council) 90

register, being struck off 103
regulations on advertising 90
GMS (General Medical Services) 64
Good Medical Practice guidance (GMC) 90
goodwill 95–7
   selling for additional an enhanced
      services 96
GP Accounts spreadsheet 40
'green socks' clause 103
growth *see* business growth

handbook, staff 26
HMRC (Her Majesty's Revenue &
   Customs) 1, 15, 60, 70, 71, 83

income 39
   breakdown 57
   nonsuperannuable 54
   superannuable 54
Institute of Chartered Accountants in
   England & Wales 44
interview
   process 21–2
   selection of candidates for 21–2
   structure 22
invoicing patients speedily 117–18, 125

job description, written 26
job satisfaction 26–7

keys to success 4

leases 13, 16
liabilities 37–40, 51, 52, 71, 85
   current 50, 69
   for debts or obligations 81–2
limited companies 2, 4, 7, 13, 60
   advantages and disadvantages 9
   forming 81–6
limited liability partnership 81–6
litigation
   patient 17, 19–20
   staff 17, 19–20, 35
loans 12, 13, 73, 74, 85, 106–9, 111, 113, 116

local enhanced services 55
locums 88

management, staff 17–35
   best practice 35
   particular issues of 24–6
   and patient problems 126
   and profitability 35
   as team 24
marketing 15
   necessity for 122–3
   to new patients 90
MDDUS (Medical and Dental Defence
   Union of Scotland) 81
MDU (Medical Defence Union) 81
meetings 11, 31
   staff 29, 35
'mini-me' phenomenon 35
mission statements 7
money as life blood of practice
   2–4, 125
mortgage 5, 6, 8, 12, 14, 64, 69, 110, 111
motivation 27
MPS (Medical Protection Society) 81

national enhanced services 55
National Insurance 88
negligence, suing for 104
net current assets 69
net profit
   per partner ratio 66, 67
   per patient ratio 65, 67
New Contract Enhanced Services 65
new contract income per patient 64–5, 67
New Contract Quality and Outcomes
   Framework 65
NHS (National Health Service) 110,
   117, 120
   and accounting 57, 63, 64, 66, 68
   and business growth 89, 91–3, 95
   and business as organism 2, 13
NHS Litigation Authority 120
nonsuperannuable income 54
nurses 10, 63, 88, 92, 93

obligations or debts, liability for 81–2
opening list to new patients 89–90
operational flowchart 81
operational model for practice 9–10
    choosing right 81–6
organism, business as 1–16
other income per patient ratio 67
overdrafts 108–9
overheads 48
overtrading 88

Pacioli, Luca 37
parity
    calculating profits 109–10
    partner joining with stages to 109
partners
    certificate 46–7
    death of 104–5
    funding retiring or deceased 104,
        105–9
    joining with stages to parity 109
        calculating parity profits 109
    request useful information from
        accounts 66–8
    sliding remuneration scale for retiring
        105
    voluntarily leaves practice 100–3
Partnership Act 1890 86, 100
partnership(s)
    advantages and disadvantages 9
    agreement 101, 125
    decision grid 8
    dissolution of 100
    forming 82–6
    as key to success 4, 7–9
    model of practice 8, 9, 16
    planning for exit from 99–111, 125
    why pay into assets of 116–17
patient(s) 115–18, 120–3
    and accounting 63, 65, 67, 68
    appealing to 15–16
    and budgeting 73, 74, 76
    and business as organism 2, 6, 10–12
    and business growth 88–90, 92–4

    as key to success 4
    litigation 19–20
    and operational model 83
    and staff 17, 24, 25, 29, 31, 32
payroll 11, 16
PCTs (primary care trusts) 2, 15
personal issues, staff 35
personal and professional development 119
    making time for 32, 125
PFI (private finance initiative) 13
planning for exit 99–111
PMS (Personal Medical Services) 64–5
post-acquisition consolidation plan 126
premises
    as key to success 4
    rent or buy? 12–15
prescriptions, theft of 30
profit 37
    allocation of 56, 102–3
    and loss account 39, 48–9, 85
    overall shares 103
    sharing 84–5, 02
profitability 3, 16, 49
    and good management 35
property capital accounts 69
publishing of company accounts 82
'Put the Practice First' 125

QOF (Quality and Outcome
    Framework) 73–5
    income 54, 65
Quickbooks 40

racial discrimination 19
recruitment, staff 11, 17, 19–22, 35, 121
    costs 63
references 22–4
    and former employers 24
reimbursements 48, 53, 63, 64
remuneration
    of partners 84
    sliding scale for retiring partner 105
    staff 36
    and staff retention 27, 35

renting or buying premises 12–15
  pros and cons 13
research, misguided or lack of, causing
    business failure 123
retirement 15, 51, 69, 89, 105, 108, 110, 111
  involuntary 103–4
  voluntary 99–103
rewarding staff 28–9

Sage 40
salaried GPs 88
salary review, annual 26
satisfaction, job 27–8
schedule of drawings 59
self-employment and business failure 124
service
  great, defining 11–12, 15
  as key to success 4
sexual discrimination 19
Shareholders Agreement 7
sliding remuneration scale for retiring
    105
solicitors 104, 120
solvency 3, 16
staff
  annual appraisal 26
  annual salary review 26
  appreciation 27
  appropriate to practice 18–19
  costs 11
  discipline 32–5
  feedback 29
  handbook, up-to-date 26, 125
  as key to success 4
  litigation 17
  management 17–35
    best practice 35
  meetings 29, 35
  motivation 27
  personal issues 35
  recruitment 19–20, 35
  retention 27, 35
    and recruitment 11
  rewarding 28–9

targets, good and bad 28
time for 31–2
training 17
treating 30–1
trust and management systems 118–19
what consitututes 10–11, 16
staff efficiency ratio 62, 63, 67
stakeholders 82
statistics, practice 61–3
subletting 12
superannuable income 54
superannuation 48, 50, 58, 60, 69, 88,
    106, 107

take-overs, practice 91–4
targets, staff
  good and bad 28
taxation 1, 9, 10, 14, 49, 57, 81, 83–5, 106,
    107, 110, 111
  accountancy and 70–1
  CGT (capital gains tax) 15
  partnership 60
  putting aside monthly income for 125
team building 28
theft 30
  of prescriptions and drugs 30
time
  giving to staff 31–2
  value of 35
treating staff 30–1
trial balance 38, 51
trusting staff and management systems
    118–19

UK Generally Accepted Accounting
    Principles 44
under-drawing 108–9

valuing partners's estate 104–5
variable vs fixed costs 79
variance analysis 79
vision, as key to success 4–6

'what if' scenarios, budgeting for 76, 79

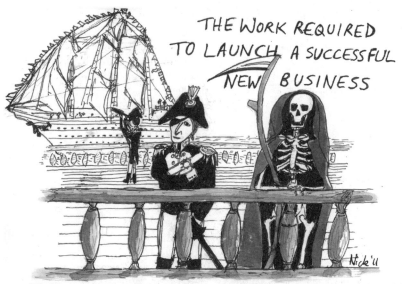

THE WORK REQUIRED TO LAUNCH A SUCCESSFUL NEW BUSINESS

IS OFTEN MUCH GREATER THAN MOST PEOPLE THINK